Yoga for Children with
Autism Spectrum Disorders

Yoga for Children with Autism Spectrum Disorders

A Step-by-Step Guide for Parents and Caregivers

Dion E. Betts and Stacey W. Betts

Forewords by Louise Goldberg and Joshua S. Betts

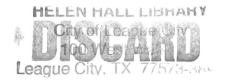

Jessica Kingsley Publishers
London and Philadelphia

First published in 2006
by Jessica Kingsley Publishers
116 Pentonville Road
London N1 9JB, UK
and
400 Market Street, Suite 400
Philadelphia, PA 19106, USA

www.jkp.com

Library of Congress Cataloging in Publication Data

Betts, Dion E. (Dion Emile), 1963-
Yoga for children with autism spectrum disorders : a step-by-step guide for parents and caregivers / Dion E.
Betts and Stacey W. Betts ; forewords by Louise Goldberg and Joshua S. Betts.
p. cm.
Includes bibliographical references.
ISBN-13: 978-1-84310-817-7 (pbk.)
ISBN-10: 1-84310-817-8 (pbk.)
1. Hatha yoga for children--Therapeutic use. 2. Autistic children--Health and hygiene. 3. Autistic
children--Rehabilitation. I. Betts, Stacey W. (Stacey Waldman), 1964- II. Title.
RJ133.7.B48 2006
613.7'046083--dc22

2006000534

British Library Cataloguing in Publication Data
A CIP catalogue record for this book is available from the British Library

ISBN-13: 978 1 84310 817 7
ISBN-10: 1 84310 817 8

Printed and bound in Great Britain by
Athenaeum Press, Gateshead, Tyne and Wear

This book is dedicated to Josh, Jake, Dan, Dora, and Sarah.
Each day with you is a treasure.

Contents

Preface   9
A note on this book   11
Foreword by Louise Goldberg   13
Foreword by Joshua S. Betts   15
Introduction   17

1: How to Use this Guide   21
Sequence of yoga poses   21
Modifications of poses and sessions   22
Demonstrate poses to your child   23
Ensure that your child is comfortable   23
A note on breathing   24
Motivating children with Autism Spectrum Disorders to practice yoga   25

**2: The Yoga Sequence for Children with Autism
       Spectrum Disorders   27**
Warm-up poses   27
    Sitting Pose   27
    Cat Pose   30
    Shoulder Opener Pose   32
    Neck Rolls   36
    Mountain Pose   39
    Spinal Rolls   41
    Chair Pose   43
Strengthening poses   45
    Triangle Pose   45
    Side Angle Pose   48
    Downward Dog Pose   51
    Warrior I Pose   54
    Warrior II Pose   55
    Standing Forward Bend Pose (A and B)   58
    Tree Pose   60
Release of tension poses   63
    Sphinx Pose   63
    Boat Pose   65
    Bridge Pose   68

Calming poses   69
    Stick Pose   70
    Seated Forward Bend Pose   71
    Spread Leg Forward Bend Pose   74
    Head-to-Knee Pose   77
    Butterfly Pose   79
    Reclining Butterfly Pose   82
    Seated Spinal Twist Pose   84
    Easy Spinal Twist Pose   85
    Child's Pose   86
    Corpse Pose   89

3: Yogic Breathing   **91**
    Ujjayi Breathing   91
    Skull Shining Breath   92
    Curled Tongue Breath   93
    Lion Breath   94
    Alternate Nostril Breathing   96

4: Shorter Yoga Sequences   **99**
    Short sequence 1   99
    Short sequence 2   100

References   *101*

Preface

We have had very profound experiences with children with Autism Spectrum Disorders. Like many parents and caregivers, we continue to search for ways of helping these children lead happy and productive lives. At the time of writing no cure for any of the Autism Spectrum Disorders has been found. In fact, no one knows for certain the cause or causes of Autism Spectrum Disorders.

Drawing on our own experiences and work with children with Autism Spectrum Disorders revealed to us that the practice of yoga can have a significant impact on the symptoms of these disorders. Why yoga?

Stacey has been practicing yoga for about ten years. From the time she was an adolescent, Stacey has been interested in ways to make her body stronger and healthier. By the time she was about twenty-seven years old, she had grown tired of typical exercise regimens that included endless repetitions including lifting weights, long aerobic classes, and expensive gyms.

Stacey discovered yoga by experimenting with a beginner yoga video. She was working as an attorney and had two small children at that time. From her first yoga session, she liked the feelings of physical strength and mental wellbeing that yoga provided. During her third pregnancy, yoga helped her to feel grounded and relaxed. Stacey expanded her practice to include more breathing techniques and intermediate poses.

Midway through her third pregnancy, our oldest son was diagnosed with Asperger Syndrome. Although the diagnosis did not come as a complete surprise, we experienced many emotions and uncertainties associated with discovering and eventually accepting that our child had a lifelong disability. Yoga helped Stacey to maintain her physical health and sense of wellbeing during that time.

As our son got older, we thought that practicing yoga could help him deal with his symptoms in a way that would not require medication, have no side effects, and be simple for him to use. Many of the yoga poses and breathing practices give individuals a sense of calm, strength, and clarity. We believed that the poses and the yogic breathing exercises could provide our son with the same benefits.

We found that yoga helps children with Autism Spectrum Disorders to reduce stress and anxiety, and increase balance and strength. We found this to be true for our son and other children with Autism Spectrum Disorders as well. This guide provides a simple approach for any parent or caregiver to use to help their children by using yoga. We believe that by using this guide, parents and caregivers of children with Autism Spectrum Disorders can help their children use yoga poses and breathing methods to lessen some of the symptoms that the children experience. No experience in yoga is needed to begin a yoga practice. It is suggested that after reviewing this guide, the reader investigate other yoga resources. A great many excellent books, videos, and other materials can help develop a deeper knowledge of yogic philosophy and practice.

A note on this book

As with any program that requires physical activity, it is advised that individuals consult a physician prior to following the program in this guide.

Foreword

I began studying yoga in earnest in 1979 when I went to Val Morin, Canada. I pitched my tent on the side of a mountain at the Sivananda Yoga Camp and lived there for the next three months. I returned each summer for six years. Swami Vishnu Devananda was the teacher at the ashram. He was extraordinarily accomplished at the asanas (yoga exercises) and well versed in the Bhagavad Gita and other yogic scriptures. He led twice daily meditations and chanting sessions, lectured on the yoga philosophy in the afternoons and evenings, and he or his teachers taught two asana and pranayama (yoga breathing) classes daily. This was a life of discipline and learning.

One of the most profound lessons Swami Vishnu offered me as a new yoga teacher was this: meet your students where they are. To me that meant that as important as it was to perform postures well, meditate, and chant Sanskrit, the most necessary qualities for a yoga teacher were non-judgment and presence. With non-judgment comes acceptance and support. With presence comes recognition and true listening. To meet a student where he is means not waiting for your student to become like you, but finding something in your yoga that speaks to your student.

This is what Stacey did with her son. And what a gift she has given him! By finding ways to make her yoga practice interesting and meaningful to her son, she has engaged him in his own practice of yoga. In now sharing that with you, she provides a foundation that may help other parents work with their own children in a similar manner. Although there is no single practice that is suitable for all children, you, too, may find something in yoga that helps your child in some way. And this is certainly worth exploring. Doing yoga is free, non-toxic, and good for you as well as your child!

Like all children, those within the autism spectrum need and deserve to be seen, heard and recognized as they are. Yoga is an excellent medium for this exchange. In my twenty-five years of teaching, I have found yoga to be a wonderful tool for children within the autism spectrum because it has the potential to meet many of their needs.

Yoga helps children build strength and flexibility. It is rare to find an exercise regime that can address both those who are floppy and those who are rigid. For every strengthening posture, there is a counter flexibility exercise. Through yoga I have seen many children within the autism spectrum improve coordination and balance. Even the most complex pose can be broken down into tiny steps, presented sequentially. Children can achieve success at many stages of the exercise.

Through yoga, dozens of the children I have taught have learned to identify tension within their bodies. Breathing exercises can help them learn to recognize when they are experiencing agitation – how that feels. In this way, parents can intervene to help children begin the slowing down process before they lose control. Even those who do not intellectualize these concepts can feel what is happening in their bodies – and yoga feels good! Relaxation feels better than tension.

There are a host of additional reasons for yoga's appeal to children within the autism spectrum. Yoga is visual. When we do yoga with children, we are physically on their level, immediately within their range of vision. We use names for postures that are very literal and recognized by most children as animals and objects from the world they know. Yoga is kinesthetic and tactile; it is immediately rewarding. The deep pressure stimulation from strengthening poses may provide relief from constant over-stimulation to the nervous system.

The language of yoga is very simple and can, in fact, be conducted without words at all. Many of the practices in yoga can be generalized to other areas of your child's life, increasing the child's independence and self-esteem. It is always a thrill to me when parents and teachers share stories of children using their yoga breath or postures at home or in school for self-calming.

Having taught yoga to hundreds of exceptional children over the past twenty years, I am convinced of its benefits. For this reason, I encourage you to select those aspects of yoga that are comfortable for you and share them with your child. There may be some things that you can do better than your child, and there may be some things that he or she can do better than you. This will be an opportunity to partner in a different way. And if you are very lucky, you may share a quiet moment together.

Louise Goldberg

Louise Goldberg is a Registered Yoga Teacher who has developed Creative Relaxation^{SM}, a program for teaching yoga based methods to children in schools. She is the author of Creative Relaxation^{SM}, Yoga for Children, a DVD featuring children within the autism spectrum. Louise has worked as a consultant to the ESE department in the Broward County Schools, Florida, since 1981, and is the owner of Relaxation Now LLC: http://www.relaxationnow.net.

Foreword: One Child's Experience with Yoga

Hello. I am one of Mom and Dad's five kids. I have Asperger Syndrome. I am eleven years old and am in sixth grade.

My mom worries about me a lot. She is always worried about how I am doing at school and how I feel. She usually wants me to feel okay. She also worries about my health. She does not want me to be too fat and she wants me to be strong. My mom will not let me eat whatever I want and she wants me to exercise my body to be healthy and strong.

My mom loves yoga. Since she loves me so much, she wants me to do yoga too. She says that yoga keeps her happy and not stressed.

I learned some yoga poses. I must say they are not as bad as I thought they would be. My body felt weird at first: very shaky and wobbly. My mom made me do this yoga stuff a lot and I actually started liking having my head upside down. I also liked when my mom told me things to think about while I was doing the poses. She told me to think about being a warrior and being brave and strong when I am doing some of the poses.

Sometimes when I am bored at school, I think about these stories to make the time go faster and to stop myself from flapping so much.

The weirdest thing my mom makes me do is breathe in strange ways.

Mom said that the breathing could help me stop flapping when I am not supposed to. I used to flap at the bus stop all the time, because I was bored and nervous about the school day. Mom told me to take some breaths and she breathed with me. Since I was thinking about my nose and air coming into my body, I could not think about flapping at the same time.

I will tell you that when I acted like a lion and did Lion Breathing, it scared all my brothers and sisters. I guess I have to say that I think yoga is weird. But, I like to spend time with my mom. Since she likes to do yoga, that is what Mom and I do together.

Joshua S. Betts

Introduction

Yoga is a practice consisting of physical postures and breathing exercises that help to unite the body and mind. Yoga originated in India many centuries ago and is gaining great popularity throughout the world. Yoga's benefits include stress reduction, inducing calm, muscle building, flexibility, and coordination. After each yoga practice, individuals simply feel better. Yoga seems to give the body what it needs.

After observing first-hand the difficulties that affect children with Autism Spectrum Disorders (ASDs), we thought yoga could provide a good basis for these children to get in touch with their bodies. We thought that we could choose yoga poses that would most meet the unique needs of children with ASDs.

Additionally, we suggest visualizations to use with most poses to help engage the mind and relax the body into the pose. The yoga postures and breathing exercises outlined in this guide were selected to address issues related to children with ASDs. Specifically, the particular sequence of the poses, and the shorter pose suggestions, were developed to allow a child with an ASD, five years of age and older, to learn a well-rounded yoga practice.

The yoga poses in this book are derived from the principles of Hatha yoga. Hatha yoga is based on helping the body to achieve homoeostasis, or a state of balance and harmony. Hatha yoga is the most common and familiar type of yoga practiced in the western world. It consists of a series of asana (poses) that emphasize alignment, breathing, and holding the body in a certain way.

There has been some medical research to show the benefits of yoga and yogic breathing. Yogic breathing has been shown to slow cardiovascular rhythms (Bernardi *et al.* 2001). Certain kinds of yogic breathing may also improve spatial memory tasks (Naveen *et al.* 1997).

Yoga may also ameliorate symptoms of asthma (Khanam *et al.* 1996). Some research suggests that yoga may be effective in treating symptoms of mental health disorders (Shannahoff-Khalsa and Beckett 1996) and in the treatment of neurological disorders (Panjwani *et al.* 1997).

Yoga has also been shown to increase the motor performance of school-children (Telles *et al.* 1993). More medical research is needed to show the physiological and mental benefits of practicing yoga.

A child with a diagnosis of an ASD shows both physical and emotional symptoms of the disorder. Children with ASDs often have low muscle tone. Muscle tone may limit your child's ability to participate in activities that require strength and endurance. Physical activity may be difficult and cause him or her to tire easily. A child with low muscle tone may not have the stamina to participate in group activities at school. Although low muscle tone may seem like a minor problem, this symptom may have a large effect on your child's mobility and confidence in joining others in a physical activity. This limitation may also impair a child's self-esteem, especially concerning athletics.

A child with an ASD often has a gross motor delay. Many children with ASDs cannot run as quickly or smoothly as other children. These kids look clumsy and awkward when they move. This awkwardness is apparent to others and often results in teasing at school. Often, children with ASDs are picked last for teams in gym class and other athletic activities.

Children with ASDs often have difficulty in reaching milestones that may not be an issue with typical children. Due to gross motor delay, low muscle tone, and the resulting impaired coordination, some kids with ASDs have difficulty learning to ride a bicycle, skateboard, or rollerblade. Not being able to do these types of activities may result in low self-esteem and lack of confidence that extend to other areas of their lives. This may also result in not wanting to do other physical activities. This sort of avoidance may result in alienation from others, and health problems like obesity.

The physical symptoms of ASDs, while seemingly slight, may drastically impair wellbeing and health. These children need an appropriate and enjoyable physical program. The practice of yoga assists individuals with both strength and balance. The poses improve strength in the large muscles of the body and may increase the tone of the muscles. Yoga poses may also help to improve balance by helping your child become aware of the placement of his or her legs and feet in relation to the rest of the body. The resulting muscle strength and balance control may improve coordination. When the poses are practiced consistently, your child will feel more comfortable in his or her body, which can carry over into other areas of their life.

Fine motor skills such as writing or cutting with scissors are also a challenge for child with an ASD. The problem of low muscle tone extends into the fingers and hands of children. Yoga emphasizes being in tune with the entire body, including the hands and fingers.

Many poses in this guide include a visualization component that increases the awareness of the entire body, from the soles of the feet up through the fingertips. The visualizations, which include the idea of opening the hands and wrists, help to increase strength and functioning of the hands and fingers.

Another prevalent feature of children with ASDs is that they have many sensory issues. For example, they are often extremely sensitive to bright lights. These children also cannot tolerate loud noise. The taste, texture, and smell of food may present a problem to them. Clothing labels may cause discomfort to a child with an ASD. Some children, when presented with such stimuli, become upset and agitated. This behavior may cause your child's peers to view him or her as different. These behaviors may lead to social isolation and feelings of loneliness.

In addition to the sensory problems discussed above, children with ASDs often "perseverate." Perseveration is a repetitive movement that seems to be uncontrollable. These movements may take the form of arm flapping, clapping, or pressing the fingers together repeatedly. Perseveration occurs when a child is agitated, bored, upset, or overwhelmed by sensory input.

Yoga may address and decrease these sensory problems in several ways. First, the physical practice of yoga soothes the nervous system. Yoga provides poses of flowing movements that allow energy to be released from the body. As your child goes through the movements of the yoga program, his or her body will become soothed and anxiety will lessen. By practicing the poses, an overburdened sensory system is calmed and quieted. Moreover, the physical poses offer a non-competitive physical activity that releases pent-up energy. By practicing yoga, your child will have a respite from his or her usual experience of a sensory overloaded body.

An important aspect of yoga is that the poses and the breathing exercises, as well as the visualization that accompanies the poses, are portable. Breathing practices are easy to learn and remember. Your child may use these exercises anywhere and anytime he or she needs to feel calm.

Furthermore, these breathing practices are quiet and will not draw attention to your child. The yogic breathing may relieve stress, release anger and pent up emotions from the body, and balance the nervous system quickly and quietly.

On an emotional level, many children with ASDs feel socially isolated from their peers. They may have difficulty in initiating and maintaining a conversation with friends. It is often difficult for them to make friends because they do not understand how to converse appropriately or to take the perspective of other individuals.

Children with ASDs often have a narrow focus of interest. This intense interest in one subject makes it difficult for a child to converse about any other topic. This conversational difficulty may manifest itself in anger, irritability and the child feeling worthless and strange. Practicing yoga may help a child feel more at peace with his or her body. Once your child is calmer and more focused, he or she may be able to concentrate better on learning social skills.

Yogic philosophy values individual differences. Each individual should accept him or herself and celebrate the differences of others. Yoga can help a child with an ASD accept his or her unique personality and behaviors. Additionally, the yoga community is comprised of understanding and compassionate individuals. It may be helpful for children with ASDs to become a part of such a community of practitioners.

1: How to Use this Guide

This guide provides a basic yoga sequence that may be used for children with Autism Spectrum Disorders (ASDs). This sequence consists of "Warm-up," "Strengthening," "Release of tension," and "Calming" poses. Your child should be encouraged to work towards practicing all of the poses.

There are several reasons why we chose this particular sequence of poses. There are many other yoga positions but these poses are particularly helpful for children with ASDs. These poses are less intimidating and not as physically demanding as other yoga poses. In spite of their simplicity, the poses are very beneficial in reducing stress, building strength, and in calming. Many modifications may be made to make these poses more comfortable.

We have attempted to make the poses as technically correct as possible, so you may understand the full, unmodified pose. Several breathing exercises are also explained. The breathing techniques may be taught and used separately from the yoga session. Separating the physical poses from the breathing techniques will help your child not be overwhelmed by instruction. In addition, the breathing techniques are very effective and can be used at any time of day, for example, during times of stress, agitation, anger, or boredom.

Finally, to simplify the text for the reader, the male gender is used when referring to your child. As an example, instead of "himself and herself," "himself" is used. You should know that yoga is equally effective for males and females.

Sequence of yoga poses

All poses may be used or you may select one or more poses from each of the following categories in this order:

1. Warm-up poses

2. Strengthening poses

3. Release of tension poses

4. Calming poses.

Modifications of poses and sessions

The sequence of yoga poses includes several ways to modify the practice to individualize each yoga session to your child's needs. Modifications in the actual physical poses are included in the description of each pose. You need to be able to assess your child's physical abilities and limitations to determine which modifications are necessary. In addition, remember that his abilities might change from day to day and from yoga session to yoga session. On any particular day, he may be less flexible than he was the day before and therefore may need a modification that was not previously used.

In the beginning sessions, watch your child carefully to determine what is needed to make the pose most comfortable and effective for him. Suggestions are given in each pose to make them easier, if necessary. The modifications are easy to do and will make the yoga session more enjoyable. Remember that yoga is not competitive, and a modification does not decrease the merit of the session or the pose.

Some poses may be modified using "yoga props." A yoga prop is a piece of equipment that makes the pose easier to do. The use of props can help your child achieve the feeling of the poses even if he is not able to do them fully. Some types of props include pillows, blocks, blankets, and stools. All of these items may be purchased from a yoga catalog, or you may initially use items found in your own home. At the start of the yoga session, gather the items that you will need.

Stools may be needed for some standing poses. The use of a stool may help your child achieve the feeling of the pose even if he is not feeling particularly strong or flexible. Any household stool that is steady is sufficient. A folded blanket is suggested to support his neck in the supine positions and his hips in the seated positions.

Eye bags may be used in some relaxation poses. Eye bags help to block out light to allow a higher level of relaxation. They are available in different colors and come either scented or unscented.

Selecting your own poses

Another modification you may try out is to select a different sequence or number of poses at first. Although the full sequence of all the poses can be your goal for your child, at first you are advised to use just a few. Suggested shorter sequences of poses are given in Chapter 4.

When you select poses, choose from each of the four categories (Warm-up poses, Strengthening poses, Release of tension poses, and Calming poses). No matter how many poses you choose, the yoga session should always end with Child's Pose and Corpse Pose, which help your child to relax, unwind, and allow his body to absorb the benefits of the session.

Demonstrate poses to your child

Verbal instruction and excessive talking may be distracting for children with ASDs. You will need to model the pose and use physical prompting, as long as your child does not react negatively to touch.

Prior to the first yoga session, talk to your child briefly about yoga and the breathing exercises. In addition, review some of the pictures of the yoga poses so he gets the general idea of yoga.

Initially, work very closely with your child to make sure that he is comfortable and stable in each pose. Until he is familiar with the selected yoga poses, demonstrate each of the poses to make them clear. Then, the pose should be done by each of you at the same time, preferably with your mats facing each other. This way your child may see how the pose is done and you may assess how he is doing.

Hands-on prompting may be needed to help your child feel comfortable and steady in the pose. In time, he will be able to use the poses and breathing exercise on his own and with much less assistance.

The poses are geared toward children age seven and above, however, younger children may also benefit. The poses would not harm any child at any age, however, from our experience, kids at about age seven begin to understand the way to come into and hold a pose.

In many of the poses, suggested visualizations are given. First, ensure that your child is comfortable and stable in the pose. You may then describe the particular visualization. At first, he may not be able to concentrate on any visualization and may feel overwhelmed with the act of achieving the pose. Additionally, he may find the sound of your voice irritating and a distraction. You will need to use discretion to determine whether or not to include the visualization in a particular pose on a particular day.

The idea of the visualization is to enhance the yoga experience, not to agitate your child. In addition, over time, you and your child may create some unique visualizations.

Ensure that your child is comfortable

Any time of day is appropriate to practice yoga. Some children like to do some poses in the morning before school, to ground them and to wake up. Others may prefer to practice yoga after school or before bed. It really is up to you and your child to determine what time of day works for your schedule. Try to be consistent with the time of day, so your child and his body are used to taking a yoga break. Before practicing yoga, have your child wait one hour after eating, so that his belly is not too full and he does not feel sluggish from digestion of food during the session.

Each participant should have a yoga mat and be in bare feet. A very popular and effective yoga mat is called a "sticky mat." The sticky mat is to help your child feel that his feet and legs are stable in the poses. He should not feel as if he will slide on the mat. Yoga catalogs have different types of sticky mats, and you should be able to find one to suit your child. There are mats made with natural fibers, if an artificial sticky mat is uncomfortable. In addition, there are different thicknesses of mats. Peruse a yoga catalog to determine which mat would be best for your child.

Your child should not wear regular socks, as this will not provide the needed stability. If he is uncomfortable on a yoga mat with bare feet, you may purchase yoga socks and open-finger yoga gloves that provide the same stability without the sticky feeling. In addition, these gloves and socks are portable and convenient if you are traveling and want to practice yoga without carrying a mat with you.

Daily practice is beneficial to help your child to become familiar with the feeling of being in yoga postures. However, if this is not feasible, yoga should be practiced at least three times a week. A yoga session only needs to be ten minutes long if done daily or a few times a week. Consistent practice will increase a child's energy level, balance, strength, stamina, and coordination.

The child should wear loose and nonbinding clothes. The fabric needs to be comfortable. The fabric should be light and loose, such as a light cotton shirt and shorts. The same outfit could be worn for each session so that your child will understand that putting on the yoga outfit means that the yoga session is about to begin.

When getting into or out of poses, your child should always move slowly, to be sure that the full pose is comfortable. The entire yoga practice should be gentle and comfortable with no excessive strain or stress. After poses are practiced, more advanced yoga positions and sequences may become appropriate. Your enthusiasm and participation in the yoga practice will be a great influence on your child to start and continue the practice of yoga.

A note on breathing

Yogic breathing involves breathing through the nose as opposed to the mouth. The beginner needs to concentrate on taking deep breaths in between poses. During the poses, breathing may be done normally at first. Eventually, your child may want to pay more attention to inhaling and exhaling during the poses. Specific breathing instructions are included in each pose description.

Yogic breathing means breathing deep down into the belly, instead of breathing shallowly into your chest. You may explain to your child that you do not want him to breath like a superhero (chest in and out). Instead, it should appear as if the belly were filling with air on inhalation and the belly should retract into the spine during exhalation, while the air is pushed out. Chapter 3 provides detailed information about breathing methods.

Motivating children with Autism Spectrum Disorders to practice yoga

As parents of a child with an ASD, we were willing to try anything we could to make our son's life better. When we first introduced the idea of yoga to our son, he balked. He refused to listen to our plans about implementing a yoga practice for him. He also did not want to hear about the positive benefits of yoga. Our son did not even want to hear the word "yoga." Even though we were convinced that yoga would help our son with the symptoms of Asperger Syndrome, we could not motivate him to try even one pose with us.

Our son thought it seemed like too much work. He viewed yoga as exercise and he knew that he was not athletic. He also thought the whole idea of yoga and paying attention to his breathing was weird. Yoga seemed to be yet one more thing that he "had" to do. He also believed that boys and men did not practice yoga and that if he practiced yoga he would be more "different" than other kids.

We realized that we needed to begin yoga very slowly with our son. We started with just one pose. We had him hold the pose for just one second. We also modified the pose for him to make him as comfortable as possible. We used modifications not normally mentioned in any other book or guide. Additionally, we listened to his complaints and changed the pose to accommodate him. He had his back rubbed while he was guided into the pose.

After our son understood and became familiar with some of the poses and the breathing techniques, he began to be less resistant to the whole process. We felt that he really succeeded when he did some breathing techniques at the bus stop independently.

We suggest that you find something that may motivate your child to try just one pose. The number of poses and the length of time that your child is in the poses is irrelevant. The benefits of these poses and the practice of yoga can stay with your child for a lifetime.

Yoga is not competitive, and frustration and anger defeat the energy that goes into the practice. If you find yourself becoming frustrated with your child during a yoga session, take a break, or continue on another day. In addition, the breathing exercises in Chapter 3 may be extremely helpful in relieving frustration.

2: The Yoga Sequence for Children with Autism Spectrum Disorders

Warm-up poses

Sitting Pose

This first pose (Figure 2.1) is used to ease into the yoga session and let your child know that the yoga session is about to begin. Because children with Autism Spectrum Disorders (ASDs) often have difficulty transitioning from one activity to another, this first pose is a consistent way to start the day's yoga practice. The pose provides a few minutes when you and your child may relax, let go of stress and worries, and prepare for the practice.

As a modification, use a firm pillow under the hips, to make your child comfortable and provide support. If your child has very tight hips or weak abdominal or low back muscles, he may not be comfortable in any type of cross-legged position, with or without a pillow. If this is the case, he may sit on a low stool to practice the seated positions in this and the following poses (see Figure 2.2). Once your child is in the pose, you may tell him to imagine that he is a Buddha: still and peaceful.

1. Begin by sitting erect at the front of your mat.

2. Cross your legs in any comfortable position. You may need a blanket under your hips for comfort in the seated position.

3. Take a moment to concentrate on how you are feeling. Listen to the sounds of your environment.

4. Close your eyes and take a deep inhalation into your belly through your nose.

5. Hold your breath and release it slowly. Contract your belly towards your spine to exhale all of the air out of your body.

6. Take this deep breath and release it three times, each time thinking about how your body feels. Be relaxed and motionless. Pay attention to how you are feeling.

7. Continue to breathe deeply through your nose and release your breath through your nose. Try to make both your inhalation and exhalation long and smooth. Breathe deeply for several moments and proceed to the next pose.

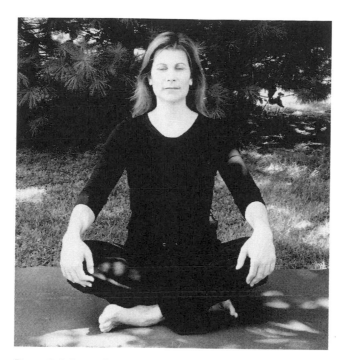

Figure 2.1 Sitting Pose

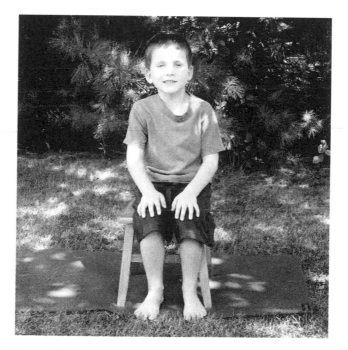

Figure 2.2 Modified Sitting Pose

Cat Pose

Cat Pose (Figure 2.3) will help make your child aware of how the movement of his body connects to his breathing. Cat Pose also helps to warm and loosen the body for subsequent poses. Specifically, the pose loosens the spine and begins to open the chest. The movement of this pose may also help digestion, as it gently massages the internal organs.

Initially, the pose may make your child's arms feel tired. If so, you may need to shorten the duration of the pose. As the name of the pose implies, the action of the body is similar to a cat stretching after a nap. Your child may imagine a cat stretching his body and spine to awaken all parts of his being. The "cat" idea may give him a good sense of the movement of this pose. You may want to tell a brief story about a cat awakening and his daily routine of stretching and moving his body to ready himself for the day ahead. As a modification, you may support the child's torso in your arms (Figure 2.4). You can do this until his abdomen and back muscles are strong enough to support himself.

1. Start in the center of the mat on your hands and knees. Position hands directly beneath your shoulders and your knees in line with your hips.

2. To bring awareness to the hands and open up the hand and wrists, fingers should be fully spread and the hands should press firmly into the mat.

3. Your neck should be relaxed and your head hanging down.

4. Take a deep breath and bring your body into a cat position. Round your back upward and tuck your tailbone down.

5. Tuck your chin down towards your chest and curl your head inward.

6. Continue to press firmly down through your hands. Try to stay lifted out of the shoulders and do not allow your shoulders to sag.

7. Hold this pose for three full breaths and then release back into the original position. Stay like this for a minute and then release and stand at the front of your mat.

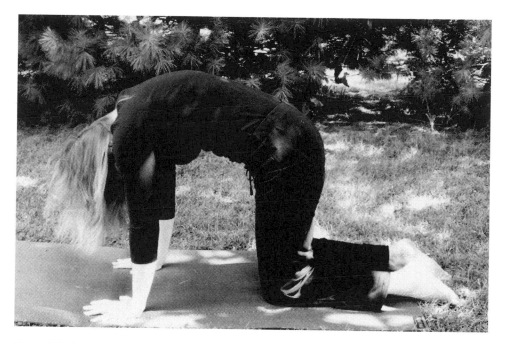

Figure 2.3 Cat Pose

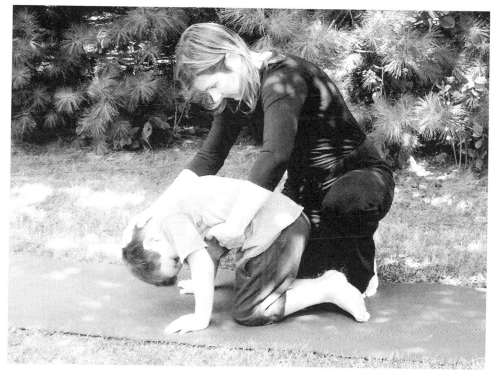

Figure 2.4 Modified Cat Pose

Shoulder Opener Pose

This pose begins to loosen and open the shoulders. This posture may help your child increase movement to the entire upper body and helps to increase the range of motion in the shoulders. Shoulder Opener Pose also releases tension in the arms, shoulder, neck, and chest. This pose may increase the air brought into the lungs and increase circulation throughout the entire body. Additionally, this pose will make your child aware of his shoulder and neck region.

Tightness in the shoulders is common. Many adults and children hold tension in their shoulders. At first, the range of motion may be limited, because this is not a position in which children normally engage. With practice, the position will become easier and feel freeing. This pose will warm the upper body and release tension.

This pose helps children with ASDs become familiar with parts of their bodies that they may have never fully felt. In addition, the breathing into shoulder tightness will help your child realize that his mind and breath may help dispel discomfort he may feel at any time.

A strap, long sock, or scarf will be needed for this pose. As a modification, the child may sit on a stool if he is uncomfortable in a cross-legged position. Additionally, his arms do not have to be spread as wide as in the full version of Shoulder Opener Pose. You should ensure that he is comfortable and that there is not too much stress on his shoulders.

Furthermore, you should ensure that he does not feel that he has to force his arms in front or back of him. Initially, he may not be able to reach behind himself. You may omit this part of the pose until his shoulders feel freer to try it. He will increase his range of motion slowly, over time.

1. Sit in a cross-legged position at the front of the mat. If necessary, a firm pillow may be placed under the buttocks to lift the hips and make the position more comfortable (Figure 2.5).

2. Hold the strap in both hands with your arms spread about as far apart as your hips. Keep your arms straight (Figure 2.6).

3. Inhale and bring your arms straight up until they are vertical from your shoulders. Feel as if you are extending your arms toward the ceiling (Figure 2.7).

4. Stay in this position for several moments, feeling the elongation of your arms upward. Your shoulders should become warm with the sustained holding of your arms upward.

5. Release your arms from holding the strap. Reach your arms behind your body and feel your chest expand (Figure 2.8).

6. Hold for several moments and allow the shoulders to release and become accustomed to this position.

7. Bring your arms overhead and in front of you to the starting position.

8. The whole movement, front to back, may be done three times. As you become used to this movement, you will be able to reach further behind your body as tightness in the shoulder area decreases. When you feel the tightness in the shoulders, inhale, and exhale deeply into the tightness. Over time, it will begin to lessen.

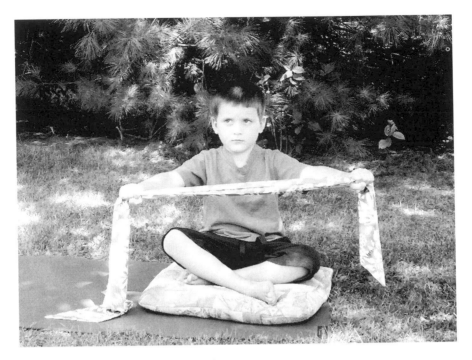

Figure 2.5 Modified Shoulder Opener Pose

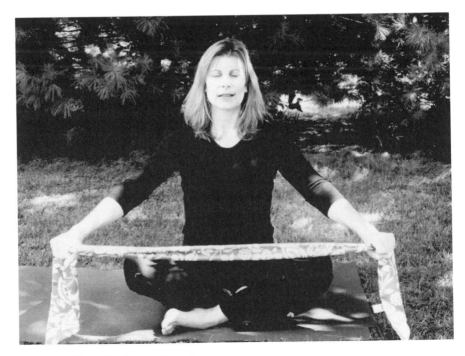

Figure 2.6 Shoulder Opener Pose A

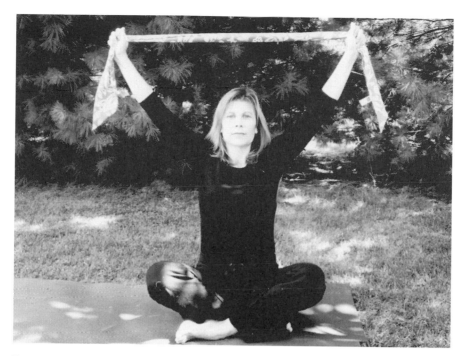

Figure 2.7 Shoulder Opener Pose B

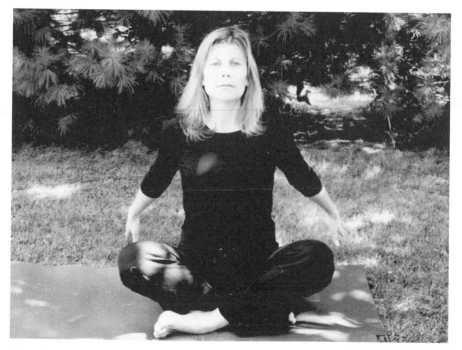

Figure 2.8 Shoulder Opener Pose C

Neck Rolls

Neck Rolls release tension and stress in the neck and face. Often, a child holds a lot of tension in these areas. Tension builds over time, leading to agitation and perseveration. This posture invigorates the neck and will help make your child aware of this area of his body. Neck Rolls is a relatively easy pose for a beginner to master. Neck Rolls are particularly effective for children with ASDs because they release tension that they may not recognize that they have.

Usually, modification of the pose is not necessary. Remember to have the child make his head move slowly and smoothly. He should not stretch his neck to the point of pain. He may visualize his head as a ripe fruit (head) on a stem (neck). Then, the fruit may gently rotate around on the stem so that all sides of the fruit are exposed to the sun.

1. Sit cross-legged at the front of your mat. Sit on a pillow or stool if necessary to elevate the hips and make you more comfortable.

2. Relax the shoulders and sit quietly.

3. Slowly begin to tilt the neck to the right, so your right ear is over your right shoulder (Figure 2.9).

4. Try to keep your shoulders down and feel the stretch on the left side of your neck. Only stretch as far as is comfortable.

5. Hold for one count and then release your head backward with your face pointed upward. Imagine your face as fruit looking toward the sun and gathering its energy. Keep your eyes closed and focus on the feeling of your throat stretching and opening (Figure 2.10).

6. Hold for a moment and then roll the head to the left, stretching out the right side of the neck. Keep your shoulders down, relax your face, and close your eyes (Figure 2.11).

7. Continue rolling your head to the right and let your head drop to your chest for a moment to stretch the back of the neck (Figure 2.12). These movements are one round of Neck Rolls.

8. Pick your head up and look straight ahead. You and your child should try to think about how your necks and heads feel. You will probably feel freedom and openness in your necks.

9. Do Neck Rolls twice more to the right, and then switch directions going to the left side. Do three Neck Rolls for this side. When finished, lift your head and stand at the front of your mat.

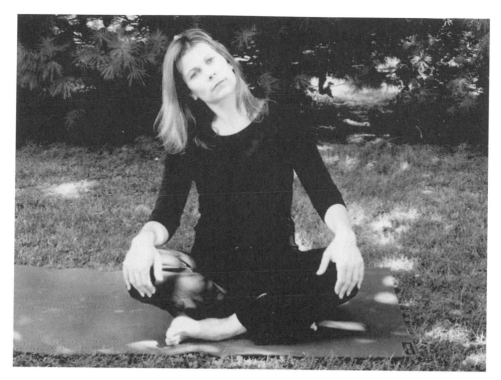

Figure 2.9 Neck Rolls A

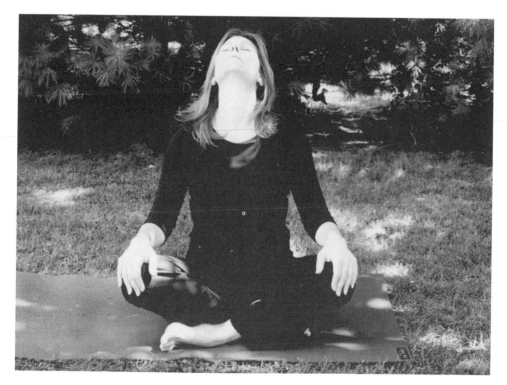

Figure 2.10 Neck Rolls B

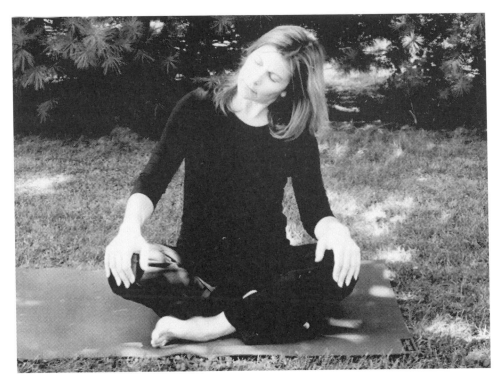

Figure 2.11 Neck Rolls C

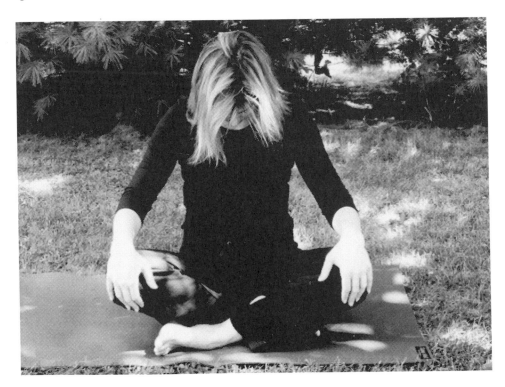

Figure 2.12 Neck Rolls D

Mountain Pose

Mountain Pose (Figure 2.13) is the first standing warm-up pose in the yoga sequence. Mountain Pose helps familiarize your child with the feeling of standing on the mat in preparation for the strengthening poses that follow. Practicing this pose will help him to feel grounded by having his legs and feet press into the floor. Mountain Pose will introduce him to the idea of the lower body pressing into the earth while the upper body and torso elongate, creating a feeling of spaciousness with stability. This pose helps to establish good posture.

This pose is not particularly physically taxing and is a very effective pose for awakening the whole body. Your child may concentrate on standing with different parts of his body lifting and grounding. You may help him visualize his head and chest lifting, while his feet and legs press downward, lengthening the spine.

A visualization may be that your child sees himself as a mountain. The mountain has two components to its stability. The mountain is very still and straight and cannot be moved by the wind or the rain. The mountain reaches to the sky and extends its base into the earth to feel and use the earth's energy, solidness, and stillness. The mountain also reaches to the sky and the sun to gain energy from the universe.

This pose helps children with ASDs become better aware of their body in relation to the environment. The pose may also help your child begin to recognize how all parts of his body feels. It may also make him aware of the amount of space that his body takes up in the environment and the boundaries and limits of his physical being.

1. Move to the front of the mat and bring your feet together so that they are touching. The toes should be spread out and the feet pressed into the mat. Your body weight should be pressing through your legs and feet into the mat. If your feet cannot touch comfortably, keep them about one foot apart (Figure 2.14).

2. Keep your arms at your sides and relaxed.

3. The shoulders should be relaxed and rolled down the back. It should feel like your chest is expanding and opening and that your rib cage is lifting.

4. Take a deep inhalation and feel your belly expand with your breath. Exhale and pull your belly inward to expel all the air out of your body.

5. Try to do this pose with your eyes closed to bring your energy from your breath inward. If it is too difficult to balance with your eyes closed, keep the eyes open and maintain a soft gaze directly facing forward. You will want to check your child's body position to make sure he is as straight as possible and relaxed.

6. Hold this pose for five breaths.

7. When you have finished the pose, relax your body and stand at the front of your mat.

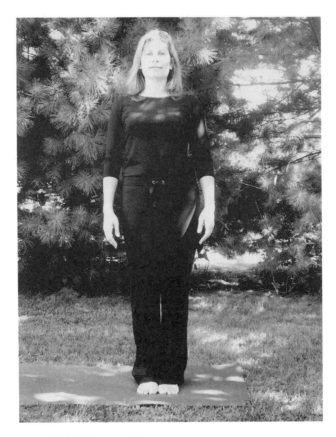

Figure 2.13 Mountain Pose

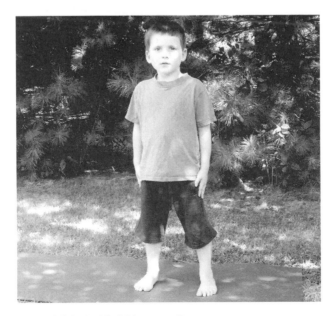

Figure 2.14 Modified Mountain Pose

Spinal Rolls

Spinal Rolls (Figure 2.15) provide a warm-up for the standing poses and continue the loosening process of the spine that was begun in the sitting poses. This pose will stretch the upper back to relieve tension in the shoulders. Spinal Rolls also warm up the hamstrings and begin to bring flexibility to the spine and legs. Even though this pose seems simple, it engages the whole body and brings awareness to the body.

A modification to the pose is to have your child roll his spine less deeply into the pose. He should only go down as far as is comfortable and then return to the original position (Figure 2.16). He is unlikely to be able to reach the floor if you are modifying the pose. He may need you to support his torso as he is rolling down into the pose. This support will help your child feel steady. As a further modification, he may only practice the pose one time during the first sessions.

This pose may be difficult although it looks deceptively easy. Encourage your child to allow his spine to loosen with each roll. He may imagine that his spine is a waterfall that cascades into the earth each time he rolls downward. Have him "see" his spine unfurling as a waterfall would flow downward, with suppleness and grace. Initially, this pose may be uncomfortable because often the entire spine is tight and compressed. Imagining a flow of water will help the mind let go of the tightness in the spine.

1. Come into Mountain Pose. Feel the entire body as being strong and steady, with the feet pressing into the floor.

2. Slowly lower the head to the chest.

3. Take several breaths and then begin to curl forward until you are hanging over your legs. Your legs may remain straight, or your knees may bend slightly.

4. When you are bent over as far as is comfortable, let your arms and head hang loosely and take several breaths.

5. To come out of the pose, press into your feet and slowly straighten the spine. Your arms should remain at your sides. Take several breaths and then begin to roll down again. This pose can be practiced three times during a session.

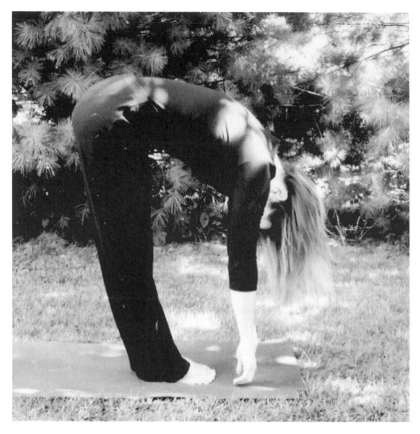

Figure 2.15 Spinal Rolls

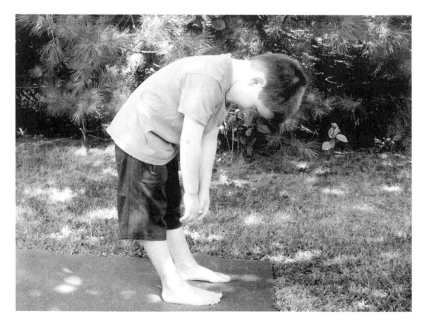

Figure 2.16 Modified Spinal Rolls

Chair Pose

Chair Pose (Figure 2.17) increases strength and endurance. It warms the body and strengthens the abdominals and thighs. This pose is a rather strenuous pose. If your child is tired, make the modifications suggested below. Even if he can hold this pose for just one breath, the pose is beneficial for the entire body. Encourage him to practice the pose, even if it is challenging.

This pose is a good leg strengthener, and enlivens and brings energy to the thighs. Chair Pose may also strengthen the abdominals and back. If your child has difficulty keeping his feet together at first, start with the feet spread apart and his arms down. After several sessions, he will gain strength and feel more comfortable with his feet closer together. His arms may still be at his sides until he feels strong enough to raise them over his head. Once the arms are raised, they may be held overhead for a very short time at first. In time, the full pose may be achieved.

A visualization that your child may use is that he is sitting in an imaginary chair. This visualization may help him "see" what each part of his body is supposed to be doing in the pose and how his body is supposed to look. Often, children also enjoy the idea that their body is like a piece of furniture and that they do not actually need a chair to sit down.

1.   Come into Mountain Pose with the feet touching. If for some reason your child is uncomfortable with his feet so close together, you may spread his feet up to one foot apart.

2.   Slowly bend your legs as if you are sitting in a chair.

3.   Only bend the knees as far as comfortable. Do not go too deep initially. The modification in this pose is to keep the knees only slightly bent until strength and comfort increase.

4.   Reach your arms upward, about shoulder width apart. If this is not possible keep your arms at your sides (Figure 2.18).

5.   Hold this pose for three full breaths.

6.   This pose may be challenging for children with low muscle tone, so your child may only be able to hold the pose for one breath or less. In time, your child may hold the pose for the full breath count.

7.   Your head may be tilted upward slightly to the sky, if that is comfortable for your neck. If not, look straight ahead.

8.   When finished with the pose, stand at the front of the mat to begin the strengthening poses.

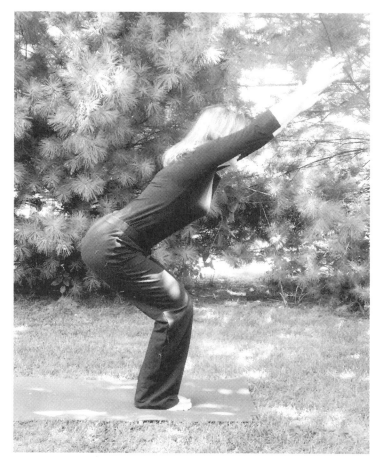

Figure 2.17 Chair Pose

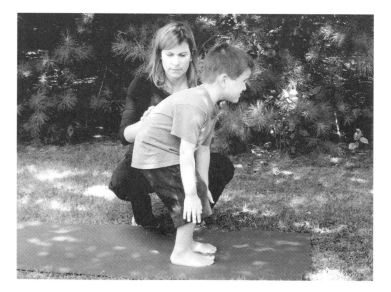

Figure 2.18 Modified Chair Pose

Strengthening poses

In general, strengthening poses are standing poses. Standing poses are poses in which your child stands on the mat with his feet spread a certain distance apart. They are named strengthening poses because they do just that. These poses strengthen and tone the large muscle groups of the body.

The muscles that are strengthened include the thighs, hamstrings, arms, and shoulders. Additionally, these poses open the hips due to the positioning of the legs. These poses also stretch the spine. Strengthening poses require some concentration and muscle strength, but they are well worth the effort.

These poses may alleviate nervous energy because they are somewhat strenuous and require the muscles to expend energy. They may also provide your child with an outlet for his excess tension.

These poses are easily accessible for a child to use when he is stressed. All your child needs to do is lay down his yoga mat almost anywhere and practice a couple of the poses. In time, he will gain strength and flexibility from these standing poses and will feel a difference in his body.

The poses that we chose are challenging enough to keep the practice interesting and stimulating, but should not overwhelm your child. In the strengthening poses, as with the warm-up poses, modifications may be made if needed. Suggested modifications are included in the descriptions of the poses. You may not want to call these poses "strengthening poses" to your child because he may feel intimidated by the idea that he needs a lot of muscle strength to do them. You may refer to these as "standing poses" and not mention that he may feel difficulty in his muscles.

Triangle Pose

Triangle Pose (Figure 2.19) is the first standing pose that strengthens the legs and opens the hips. It also lengthens the torso and the spine. Over time, Triangle Pose may increase flexibility of the entire body, and increase strength in the lower body. This pose may also bring a feeling of lightness and openness to the entire body. Your child is taught to think about his legs pushing into the floor while his arm is reaching toward the ceiling.

Children with ASDs sometimes have difficulty orienting their body to the environment. Triangle Pose, with the arms and legs reaching from the torso, makes your child begin to be aware of his body space in the external environment. This pose also helps to open the chest allowing for deeper breathing.

Triangle Pose may look intimidating. You will need to guide your child into the pose initially, as opposed to only modeling the pose. You may need to help extend his arm upward as he may not have the arm strength to do this independently. Additionally, you may use a stool as a modification until he gains flexibility in the hips and legs. You can have your child visualize their body looking like a triangle. You may then demonstrate the pose to show how the body does look like a triangle. He may become so interested in how he may "look like a triangle" that he will concentrate on this image instead of any fatigue he may feel in his muscles.

In addition, you can instruct him to think about his legs pressing into the earth and his arms extending to the sky. Using these muscles will help him remain stable and strong in the torso to maintain balance.

1. Begin in Mountain Pose at the front of the mat and take a deep inhalation and exhalation.

2. Turn on the mat, spreading your legs about three feet apart. Your feet should point straight ahead and should be in a straight line.

3. Turn your right foot out ninety degrees and your left foot in about forty-five degrees. The arch of your left foot should be in line with your right heel.

4. Extend your arms out to the sides at about shoulder height. Reach strongly through the arms.

5. Keeping your legs straight, slowly begin to bend forward over your right thigh while reaching your right hand to your knee, shin, and ankle. Over time, as you gain flexibility, you will be able to extend your right hand further down the right leg.

6. As a modification, reach your right hand to a stool positioned at your side to lean on.

7. Reach your left hand to the sky and feel your arm stretch upward. Feel your chest expand and open.

8. You may relax your neck and look forward. Or, if it feels comfortable for you, slowly begin to look upwards towards your left hand. As you inhale, think about pushing through your legs and pushing your feet into the floor. As you exhale, think about stretching your left hand to the sky.

9. Hold this position for three to five breaths. As a modification, your child my hold the pose for as little as one breath. He will still feel the benefits of the pose.

10. To come out of the pose, use your legs for strength and bring your body upright. Slowly put your arms down. Keeping your feet spread apart, take a deep inhalation and exhalation (cleansing breath). Repeat the entire pose on the left side.

11. When finished, step back into Mountain Pose.

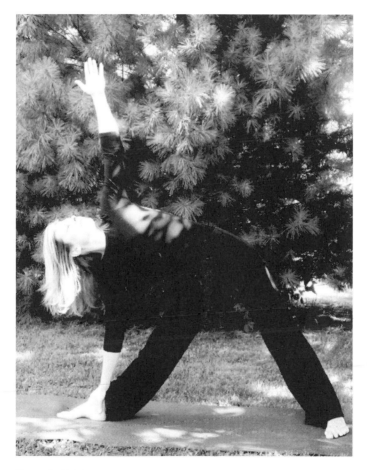

Figure 2.19 Triangle Pose

Side Angle Pose

Side Angle Pose (Figure 2.20) is similar to Triangle Pose in that it involves a similar leg stance. Like Triangle Pose, the pose strengthens the legs and opens the hips. However, in this pose the strengthening is concentrated in the thigh area.

Children with ASDs often have difficulty with competitive sports. These children need to find a physical way to release anxiety and stress. A fundamental idea of yoga is that practicing yoga should not cause mental or physical stress. When practicing yoga, your child does not have to worry about keeping up with others.

Strengthening poses provide muscle toning in an environment that is relaxing and noncompetitive. Since Side Angle Pose uses the large muscles of the leg it helps to release accumulated tension in these muscles and in the rest of the body.

Correct positioning is the key for this pose to yield desired benefits. Your child will probably need a lot of encouragement because the pose requires effort and strength, more than with most other poses. You may make modifications such as holding the pose for a shorter period or decreasing the angle of the bent leg. This will make the pose more comfortable for your child until his strength increases. You may use him as a guide to let you know when he begins to feel uncomfortable. When beginning to teach him this pose, you may have him hold the pose for as short a period as only one second.

Depending on his muscle strength, he may have to build up to this pose gradually. He should be able to feel his strength and endurance increase each time he practices. He may feel a sense of accomplishment that will carry over into other areas of his life.

He can visualize his legs pressing into the ground and his arm extending into the sky. You can tell him to "see" his arm as a strong arrow pointing into the sky. He can imagine energy coming from the ground, through his legs and up through his arms and fingers and his fingers shooting a glow of energy into the sky.

1. Start in Mountain Pose and take a deep breath.

2. Spread your feet out (about one leg length).

3. Keep your heels along an imaginary straight line.

4. Turn your right foot out about ninety degrees and left foot in about forty-five degrees.

5. Align your right heel with your left foot arch.

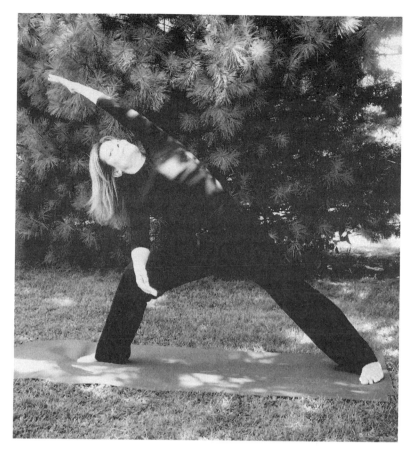

Figure 2.20 Side Angle Pose

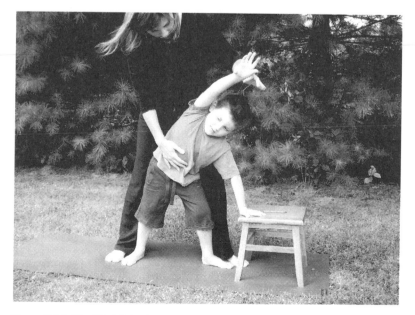

Figure 2.21 Modified Side Angle Pose

6. Raise your arms out to the side until they are at even height with your shoulders.

7. Slowly bend your right knee until it is as close to ninety degrees as possible. Your child may only be able to bend the knee a little. The benefit of the pose is not from how far the knee is bent.

8. Try to make the left leg and foot press into the floor so it may take some of the weight off the body and relieve pressure on the right leg.

9. Both feet should feel grounded into the floor and the legs should feel strong. Often, there is an intense feeling in the forward leg, where the muscles are really working. Make sure to keep your breathing deep and slow and try to breathe into the intense feeling of the leg.

10. Bend your right forearm and place it on the bent right leg. Try to keep your chest rolled open and not turned down towards your legs.

11. If it is too difficult to put your forearm on your thigh, you can place your forearm on a stool (Figure 2.21). This will relieve some of the weight from your front leg.

12. Your left hand may remain resting on your left hip during initial sessions. Over time, you will want to raise your left arm above your left ear for the full pose.

13. You may look either down to the mat to release your neck, or gaze upward toward your left arm, if this is comfortable.

14. Maintain the pose for one or two breaths during initial sessions, increasing to five full breaths over time.

15. When finished with this side, drop your arms, straighten your legs, and take a deep breath.

16. Point your feet to the left and perform the pose on the left side.

Downward Dog Pose

Downward Dog (Figure 2.22) is an inversion pose in which the hips are above the heart. This pose increases the blood flow and circulation to the heart. In this pose, the shoulders and arms become both strengthened and opened. The neck is relaxed and hanging, so any tension in the neck is alleviated. The heels are pressing towards the floor and the hamstrings are stretched and elongated. Also, the abdominal muscles are used to stabilize the torso.

This pose requires both arm and leg strength, so it may be difficult for your child at first. However, the pose is beneficial no matter how long it is held, so he should be encouraged to practice this pose and it will gradually become easier.

As the head is hanging upside down, this pose offers him a different view of his environment. You may mention that he should observe how he feels with his head upside down. He can also think about how the world looks in this position.

The positioning of the body in this pose may help a child with ASD, who may be very rigid and restricted about his surroundings, to experiment and become more comfortable with seeing his environment in a different way.

Your child can imagine himself as a dog, stretching awake. He can envision his legs reaching into the ground and his spine and tailbone lengthening into the sky. Although this pose is demanding, his visualization of himself as a dog may help to make the pose more enjoyable.

Your child should be encouraged and praised in this pose and the other strengthening poses to follow, as these poses require perseverance. Once mastered, he will feel a sense of accomplishment. In addition, the physical challenges of these poses will reduce anxiety and help him expend excess nervous energy.

1. Lay on your belly on your mat and have your arms relaxed by your sides. Legs should be relaxed and head may be turned to the side. Take several breaths before beginning the pose.

2. Put your palms under your shoulders with your elbows pointing up. Make sure the whole hand is pressing into the mat.

3. Take a breath and push into Downward Dog. Push your hips into the air. Your heels should be pressing down toward the mat. Do not worry if your heels do not generally press into the mat. Most people do not have a lot of flexibility in the calves when beginning to practice this pose. The flexibility will build over time.

4. Your abdomen should be firm to help support your torso. Try not to sink into your shoulders or let your lower back sag. There should be a straight line from the hips to the shoulders.

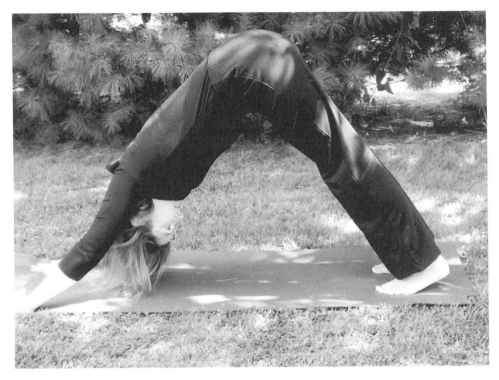

Figure 2.22 Downward Dog Pose

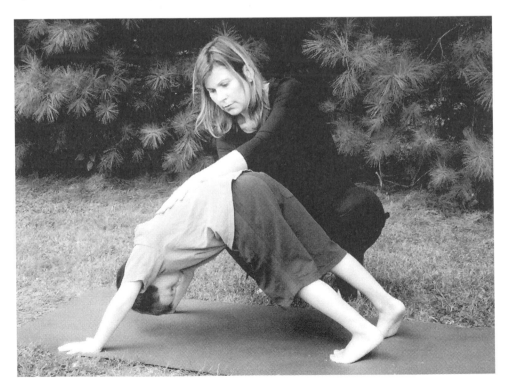

Figure 2.23 Modified Downward Dog Pose

5. Press your hands into the mat to strengthen the arms. Keep the weight of the body even between the legs and arms.

6. Hold for three to five breaths.

7. As a modification, your child may need you to support his torso until strength is gained (Figure 2.23). In addition, your child may only be able to hold the pose briefly. The idea is to get your child used to the feeling of his body in the pose. The length of time in the pose is not important.

8. After finishing the pose, come down onto the mat on your belly and rest for a breath. Come into Mountain Pose at the front of the mat to prepare for the next pose.

Warrior I Pose

Warrior I (Figure 2.24) is a pose that generates a lot of heat and energy through the entire body. The legs are rooted into the ground and the energy is brought upwards through the arms. When performing Warrior I Pose, your child may be taught to think of himself as a fierce warrior, ready to bravely face any challenge or battle encountered.

On a physical level, this pose increases strength through the legs. It also opens the hips and may release a lot of energy that is held in the groin area. By reaching to the sky, the arms and shoulders are strengthened.

On an emotional level, your child's visualization as a warrior may increase his confidence. Once he is able to hold the pose for even a short period and begins to see himself as a warrior, he may begin to feel inner strength and success. This sense of accomplishment is important to a child with an ASD. Often they have physical limitations in strength, agility, or endurance that may make them feel like a failure during typical physical activities such as sports.

Your child can imagine himself as a fierce strong warrior who can face any challenge with bravery and ease. He can internalize the idea that he is a competent and unafraid challenger. He can also envision himself conquering foes and being a hero in general. Remind him that he should remember this pose when facing obstacles in life. He may summon the strength of the warrior at any time.

1. Stand at the front of the mat in Mountain Pose and take several deep breaths.

2. Turn on the mat and bring your legs about one leg's length distance apart. Turn your right foot out ninety degrees and your left foot in about forty-five degrees. Your right heel should be in line with your left foot arch.

3. Bend your right knee as deeply as possible to ninety degrees. As a modification, only bend the knee as far as is comfortable, even if it is only a slight bend. Bending the knee deeper will require leg strength, especially in the thigh area. This strength will build over time.

4. Keep the left foot rooted into the ground and be sure to press the whole foot into the mat to support the left leg as well as the whole body.

5. Raise your arms overhead, keeping them as straight as possible. The hands may remain shoulder distance apart or they may touch, whichever is most comfortable for your child. He should imagine a powerful force being brought up through his body and out of his hands. His hands and fingers should remain spread, to get energy and circulation through the hands and wrists. As a modification, the arms can remain at his sides until your child feels capable of raising his arms overhead.

6. The belly should be firm to help support the torso.

7. Take three to five breaths in this position and then lower the arms, straighten the legs and pivot the feet to the left. Repeat the pose on the left side and then come back into Mountain Pose at the front of your mat.

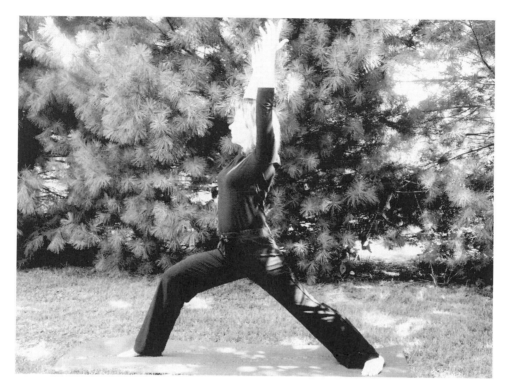

Figure 2.24 Warrior I Pose

Warrior II Pose

Warrior II Pose (Figure 2.25) has the same fierce leg stance as Warrior I but the arms are outstretched to the sides. The same leg strength is necessary for this pose, so your child will likely need some modifications initially. Although the pose is similar to Warrior I, your child should be encouraged not to skip this pose, because the feeling of freedom in the outstretched arms will invigorate him. However, if he absolutely cannot summon the strength to practice Warrior II in the beginning of his yoga practice, Child's Pose (see Calming poses) may be practiced, in order for him to rest for a few moments, before going onto the next pose.

You will need to judge how tired your child becomes while doing the poses. He may be encouraged, but not pushed beyond his endurance limit. Endurance will increase over time and does not need to be rushed, as yoga is something that may be practiced over a lifetime.

Your child can imagine being a warrior again, but this time with a specific goal in mind as he looks straight ahead past his outstretched arms. He can imagine conquering a fear as he directs his energy forward past his fingers. In addition, he can imagine the energy from the sun and sky pouring into his open chest.

He can also think about his arms extending out to the sides of the room, so he feels that he takes up a lot of space. It is important that children with ASDs feel that they are as important and worthwhile as children who do not have a disability. This pose may help a child understand that he takes up as much space, both physically and emotionally, as anyone else. His needs are as important as anyone's.

1. Come to the front of the mat in Mountain Pose and take a deep breath or two.

2. Spread your legs out on the mat about one leg's length distance apart. Turn your right foot out ninety degrees and your left foot in about forty-five degrees. Your right heel should be in line with your left arch.

3. Bend your right knee up to ninety degrees. Again, the knee should be bent only as far as comfortable, as this position requires much leg strength.

4. Press through the heels and balls of both feet to ground the body and the legs. Additionally, concentrate on putting some of your body weight on your back leg to take some of the weight off your front leg.

5. Your torso should be straight and strong.

6. Raise your arms out shoulder height and imagine that energy is coming through your arms to the front and back of the room. If your child cannot raise and hold his arms for any length of time, have him hold his arms outstretched for one second (Figure 2.26).

7. Look straight ahead and maintain a fierce gaze in front of you. Hold the position for three to five breaths and then drop your arms to your sides, straighten your legs and pivot your feet to the left side. Repeat Warrior II to the left.

8. Come out of the pose and stand at the front of your mat.

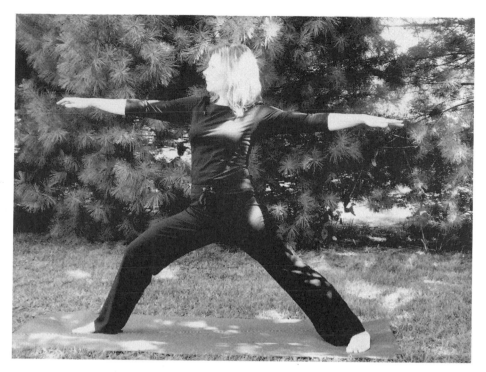

Figure 2.25 Warrior II Pose

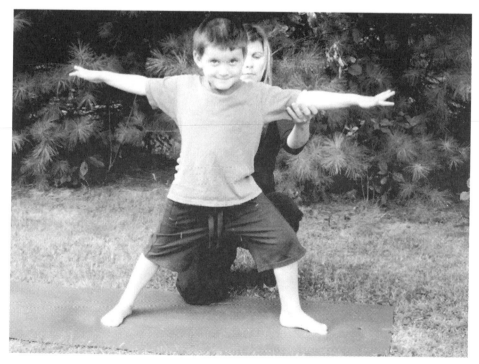

Figure 2.26 Modified Warrior II Pose

Standing Forward Bend Pose (A and B)

Standing Forward Bend Poses help to bring flexibility to the hamstrings. These poses also open the hips and stretch out the back. Two versions of Standing Forward Bend Pose may be practiced. Both versions have the same leg stance. However, the arm position is different to give the body a slightly different stretch in each pose. Both poses will strengthen the legs. Additionally, the neck will be stretched and relaxed.

Your child may have difficulty with the concept that his head will be hanging upside down. He may not like the perspective that he gets when he opens his eyes and looks around while his head is hanging between his legs. You may explain that this is a safe way to move his body and that hanging his head upside down is beneficial for his brain. The body supplies extra blood and oxygen to the brain when the head is positioned in this way.

In addition, your child can be told that it is good to allow the neck a few moments of relaxation in this pose, because the neck is usually not able to fully relax. It is to be hoped that he will understand the benefits of this pose and will accept the feeling of his head hanging upside down. You may explain that it is good to see the world in a different way and from a different perspective at times, and that this pose can remind him that seeing things upside down sometimes is both fun and necessary.

STANDING FORWARD BEND POSE A (FIGURE 2.27)

1. Turn sideways on your mat and spread your feet about three feet apart. Feet should be parallel and the feet should be pressing into the mat.

2. Firm your thighs and reach your arms out to the sides to shoulder height. Take a deep breath and feel your chest expand.

3. Slowly bend forward from the waist and place your hands flat on the ground directly under your shoulders. Let your head hang freely. Do not tense the neck or look forward.

4. If possible, bend your elbows to get a deeper stretch in the legs. If you cannot bend your elbows, keep your arms straight and take several deep breaths.

5. If you cannot reach the floor, you may rest your hands on a stool until your flexibility increases.

6. As an additional modification, if you are still uncomfortable or feel anxious in this pose, bring your feet further together so there is less of a stretch in the legs. In addition, if your child does not feel stable, you can support his torso with your hands until he feels strong enough to stand independently.

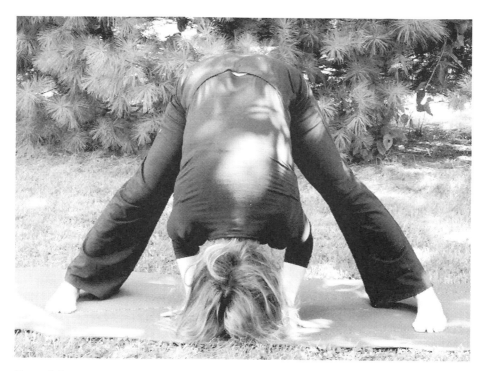

Figure 2.27 Standing Forward Bend Pose A

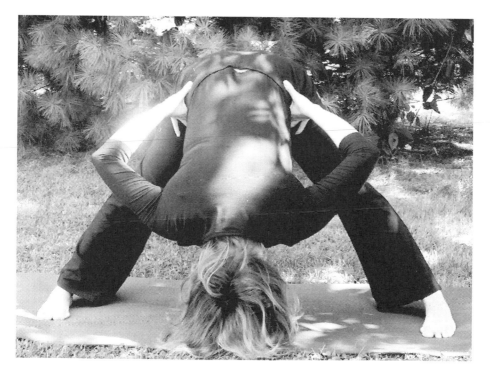

Figure 2.28 Standing Forward Bend Pose B

7.   Using the strength in your abdominals and back, keep the spine as straight as possible, and come up to a standing position.

STANDING FORWARD BEND POSE B (FIGURE 2.28)

1.   After finishing in Standing Forward Bend A, keep the same leg stance and spread your arms out to the side at shoulder height. Take a deep breath and feel your chest expand.

2.   Firm your thighs so you feel steady and place your hands on your hips.

3.   Begin to bend slowly forward from the waist, keeping your hands on your hips.

4.   When you have bent as far as possible for you, relax your neck and take three deep breaths. It is best if you keep your abdomen firm to provide support for the torso. You should feel your legs working strongly, while your upper body remains relaxed.

5.   As a modification, you can keep the legs closer together. In addition, as in Standing Forward Bend A, you can support your child's torso until he feels stable.

6.   When you are finished with your breaths, press your feet strongly into the ground and come up to a standing position.

7.   Spread your arms out to the side one last time, take a breath, and then come into Mountain Pose at the front of your mat.

Tree Pose

Tree Pose (Figure 2.29) is a balancing pose that continues to strengthen the legs. After coming into the pose, the idea is to find a point in front of you and gaze at this point, to help you maintain your balance. This pose requires concentration, and can help a child with an ASD learn to focus and connect to his body. The pose itself is not too physically challenging for most children. However, the balancing aspect usually produces some anxiety.

Your child may be afraid he will fall and get hurt. He may not want to take the time and mental focus necessary to try to balance. As with the previous poses, the benefit to the pose is in the attempt as well as the length of time that the pose is held, so proceed slowly and encourage him. Eventually he will gain balance.

Additionally, reassure him that lots of people fall initially in this pose. He will not get hurt if he loses his balance. If he is receptive, you may point out that practicing Tree Pose is a lot like life. Sometimes you will fall, but the important thing

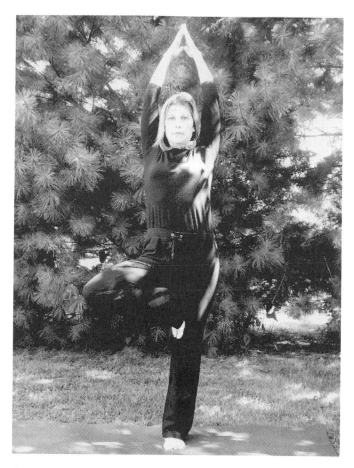

Figure 2.29 Tree Pose

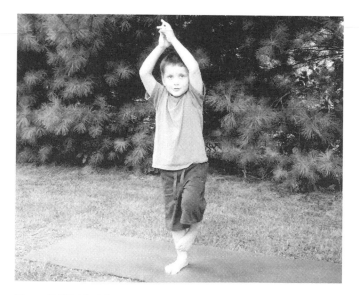

Figure 2.30 Modified Tree Pose

is to keep getting up until you are successful. Your child can be instructed to think of an image of a tree when coming into this pose. He may worry about falling down, getting hurt, and being embarrassed and feeling stupid because he fell. Reassure him that he is safe.

He may envision himself bending like a tree to try to keep balanced. However, if he does fall, remind him that falling is something that all people do at some time in their life and is not a cause for embarrassment.

1. Come to the front of the mat in Mountain Pose and take a deep breath.

2. Keeping yourself as straight as possible, bend the right leg and place the foot as high on the thigh as possible. Your entire foot should be pressing into your left leg.

3. As a modification, if you cannot bring your foot onto your thigh, bring your foot near your knee. If even this movement is impossible, keep the feet in Mountain Pose and continue to step four.

4. Slowly raise your arms over your head and gaze softly forward, maintaining your balance. If possible, your hands should be touching, with the fingers and thumb interlaced and the index fingers touching and pointing towards the sky. If you cannot touch your hands together, keep them shoulder width apart over your head. Keep your torso steady and elongate your arms to the sky (Figure 2.30).

5. If you cannot raise your arms over your head, concentrate on balancing using your legs. Leave your arms at your sides.

6. Try to maintain your balance by gazing at a point in front of you. If possible, hold this pose for three breaths. If you fall, you may try again. Do not feel too concerned if you cannot balance. Balancing is a skill that may be learned over time.

7. After you are finished with the right side, bring your leg down and then release your arms to your sides. Repeat on the other side.

Release of tension poses

These three poses are beginner backbends. These backbends are not very deep or intense, but they will help your child become familiar with the feeling of backbends. These backbends will both invigorate and calm him.

Back bending is a physical motion that is relatively unfamiliar to the body. Therefore, backbends may give him a different perspective of his body and his environment, because his body is positioned in a different way than usual.

Backbends help to relieve stress and tension in the lower back. They also help to open the entire front of the body, from the abdomen up into the chest and shoulders. Backbends may also open the throat and neck area. By opening and awakening the areas of the body that are often ignored, your child may relieve tension and stress.

Children with ASDs may be especially resistant to these poses, as they are probably more unfamiliar body positions than the previous yoga poses. Your child will likely experience anxiety during these poses. This anxiety is a sign that the poses are exposing unfamiliar areas. Tell him that this anxiety or worry is natural and acceptable. Also, tell him that the anxiety is the body's way of letting go of stress. In a short time, these feelings will lessen.

The names of the poses, Sphinx, Boat, and Bridge may help your child visualize what the poses look like, so the poses may be a little less intimidating. In addition, although these poses are effective in opening the front of the body and both invigorating and relieving tension, they do not require a tremendous amount of strength or flexibility and are accessible to most children.

As with the strengthening poses, at first, your child may not be able to hold the pose for three to five breaths. He will need to become familiar in body positions in which he has never been. These poses should not be rushed. Allow him to feel his way into each pose and to get comfortable with sensations that he may have not felt before.

As many children with ASDs can be somewhat rigid and fearful of new things, such as new physical sensations, these backbends may allow your child to experiment with feelings in his body in a new way in a safe and controlled setting. Once your child has gained confidence by experimenting with his body in a new way, he may feel more comfortable in trying other sports or physical activities.

In between these poses, Child's Pose is recommended to release the spine and provide a brief rest.

Sphinx Pose

Sphinx Pose (Figure 2.31) is the first back bending pose. It begins to open the chest slightly. It will also get your child used to the feeling of back bending. The arms extend in front of the body, rather than upwards, so the opening of the chest does not feel extreme. The idea is that the spine and chest are elongated and opened. It is important to make sure that your child is not compressing his lower back as he opens his chest. Additionally, the neck should not be bent backward. Rather, the head should face forward to get a long opening in the neck.

This pose is helpful for children with ASDs for several reasons. First, on a physical level, the back bending helps individuals lessen tension in the back, shoulders, and neck. It also stretches muscles that are normally not used, thus strengthening and releasing these muscles.

On an emotional level, as with other poses, this pose helps your child experiment with new physical sensations in a comfortable and secure environment. As children with ASDs are often resistant to change, this pose may help your child begin to learn that change and doing new activities may be fun and feel good. Additionally, your child may learn that although the new circumstance may feel intimidating, once your child is brave enough to try, the experience may begin to feel comfortable.

Children can understand the idea of being like a sphinx in this pose. We usually do not explain the idea of back bending to children because it may be too overwhelming for them to understand. Even adults who have practiced yoga for quite a while have difficulty with backbends because the movement is different and foreign and feels unnatural when it is first practiced.

You may tell your child that his head should be straight and comfortable and that he should gaze softly ahead, like a sphinx. Let him know that the sphinx is serene yet powerful and that is how he can think of himself in this pose.

1.   Come onto your belly on your mat. Your body should be relaxed and your arms should be by your side.

2.   Place your arms, palms down, about one foot in front of your shoulders.

3.   Keeping your forearms pressing into the mat, slowly raise your head and shoulders off the mat as far as is comfortable.

4.   Your gaze should be straight ahead and not upward.

5.   Your legs should be straight behind you, with your ankles together. If this is uncomfortable, allow your legs to be up to eight inches apart.

6.   You may concentrate on lifting out of the spine and the chest. The idea is to open the upper chest and back. Your child may visualize his heart coming out of a cave as his chest expands.

7.   Your breathing should be smooth and deep. Stay in this position for three breaths and come down onto your belly to release the pose. Then, come into Child's Pose for a few breaths before going into the next pose.

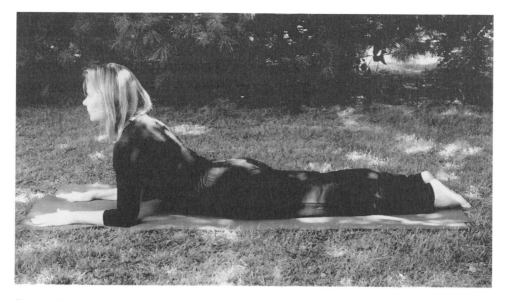

Figure 2.31 Sphinx Pose

Boat Pose

Boat Pose (Figure 2.32) strengthens the upper and lower back muscles. It also opens the chest and continues the back bending process begun in Sphinx Pose. More muscle strength is needed in Boat Pose than Sphinx Pose. It may take your child a while to be able to lift his chest and legs off the floor.

This pose will get your child familiar with using the back muscles, so the amount of height that he achieves in the pose is not relevant. This pose will release tension that is accumulated in the spine and shoulders.

Boat Pose, like Sphinx Pose, may cause anxiety at first because it exposes the chest and heart, and may cause many emotions to arise. You may explain to him that feelings of anxiety or fear are common when doing backbends, but that the anxiety will lessen as the body gets more used to moving in this way.

This pose is also a good way to demonstrate to your child that the body is very adaptable. Through these and other poses, as the body becomes familiar with moving in previously unfamiliar ways, your child can learn to control both the physical and emotional aspects of his body. This realization may help him learn techniques to help with his symptoms throughout the day.

At first, it is hard for many children to get their heads or legs off the floor. Sometimes they can just clasp their arms behind them and try to lift themselves up without being able to lift their head and legs. They are sometimes discouraged. Let your child know that this pose can be difficult. Additionally, you can tell him that any amount of lifting would "get his boat out of the water" and his arms clasping behind him is like raising the "boat" enough to keep it afloat.

The boat image helps children to visualize what movement their bodies are supposed to make. Children with ASDs make progress in this pose, which is encouraging because many have low muscle tone in their lower back and abdominal muscles. Tell your child that it is important in this pose to keep trying and practicing it consistently. He will then feel results that he may have never expected.

1. Lay on your belly with your arms by your sides and your body relaxed. Take a deep breath.

2. Clasp your hands behind your back and feel your shoulders begin to lift off the floor.

3. Gently pull your clasped hands back toward your buttocks and raise your chest off the floor. You will feel your back muscles all along your spine being used.

4. At the same time, extend your legs out from the body and raise them off the floor. The lift of the legs does not have to be high. Your child should be told to visualize his legs reaching to the back wall.

5. The legs should be as close together as possible. If this is uncomfortable, leave your legs apart, but not more than one foot apart.

6. Lifting the arms and legs should occur simultaneously. However, if your child is not strong enough to do this at first, have him lift his arms toward his buttocks and let his legs stay on the floor (Figure 2.33).

7. Try to hold the pose for three breaths.

8. Release and then rest in Child's Pose.

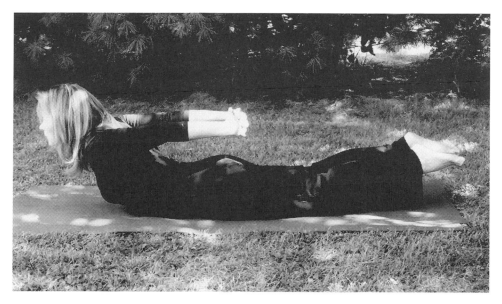

Figure 2.32 Boat Pose

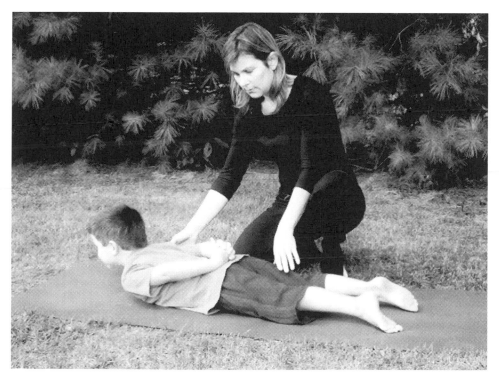

Figure 2.33 Modified Boat Pose

Bridge Pose

Bridge Pose (Figure 2.34) is a backbend that also strengthens the thighs. Your child may only be able to raise his hips a little at the beginning of the practice, but as strength and flexibility increase, the pose will get easier. This backbend also exposes the chest and heart to the sky. He may be instructed to think about his worries and anxiety floating out of his body through his uplifted chest.

There should not be strain on any part of the body in this pose. However, the legs will feel like they are being exercised. This pose helps children with ASDs to get in touch with the chest and heart. It also relieves tension. The hard work of the legs may help to expel excess energy and anxiety.

Children can benefit from seeing themselves as a bridge that has to be very strong to hold up the cars and trucks that roll over them. The vehicle idea usually provides them with enough encouragement to perform this pose. If your child does not respond to the vehicle visualization, you should try to think of another bridge-related idea. In this pose, visualization seems to help children hold the pose for a longer period.

Your child's legs may get tired quickly. We suggest that you encourage him not to collapse. If necessary, you may support his torso with your arms until he is familiar and comfortable with the pose. We are often pleased at the enthusiasm that children show for practicing this pose.

1. Lay on your back on the mat with your arms by your sides and take a deep breath.

2. Bend your knees and push your feet firmly into the ground.

3. Touch your feet with your hands. This is where your feet should remain. Your feet should be about a foot apart.

4. Leaving your arms at your sides and pushing down into your feet, slowly begin to raise your hips to the sky.

5. Roll your shoulders under and begin to lift your chest toward your chin, as your hips rise into the air.

6. As your chest is being lifted, you may clasp your hands together underneath your hips to help further raise your hips and chest.

7. Make sure your shoulders are rolling under, as this movement will bring more opening to your chest.

8. Take three deep breaths in this pose. Think about your feet pressing firmly into the floor, the strength of your thighs lifting the hips, and your chest rising to the sky. Come down slowly and lie on your back for a couple of moments to let your body absorb the benefits of back bending poses.

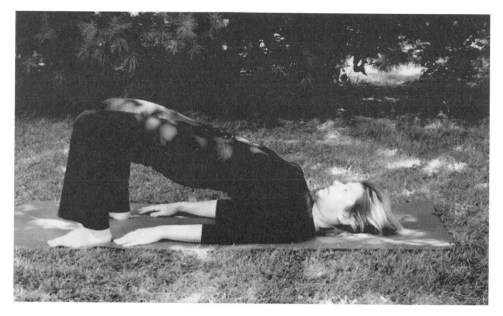

Figure 2.34 Bridge Pose

Calming poses

These calming poses are seated poses. The poses feel rejuvenating and the body does not leave the foundation of the mat and the earth. While it is true that these poses do not require much muscle strength in the extremities of the body, they are important because they both increase flexibility and calm the body. Note that these poses may be challenging to a child with an ASD, even though a great deal of muscle strength is not necessary to perform them.

As with any pose, when the body is first put into a position that it is not used to, the result may be discomfort. Calming poses should never be pushed. There may also be discomfort and even trembling as the body releases tension and anxiety and becomes more supple and yielding.

Encourage the holding of the poses for three breaths to release and soften the tissues in the body. Flexibility is not a goal in itself. Rather, it is important that there is a gradual relaxing and releasing of tension in the body.

Stick Pose

This is the first seated pose (Figure 2.35) and it is not too strenuous. It is a very effective pose for getting your child in touch with his body. This pose will lift and open the chest, firm the legs, and align the spine. It helps him to feel centered and restful, although it is an active pose. It is important to keep the arms pressing down into the mat and to keep the feet active to bring energy into the pose. Children often have difficulty in believing this is actually an active pose.

In practicing this pose, often children just want to hunch over themselves. We suggest explaining that your child should be like a stick: straight and tall. We also suggest telling your child that the body should be working hard at being aware, awake, and alive, even though it may look like the body is at rest. Since they may have low muscle tone, children with ASDs are often not very comfortable sitting in Stick Pose. Therefore, do not expect your child to hold the pose for too long. Be careful not to expect your child to be able to hold this or any other position that to you, may seem effortless. In yoga, all poses, even the still ones, require effort.

1. Come onto the back of your mat in a seated position.

2. Stretch your legs out in front of you. The feet should be flexed and the legs should be firm.

3. Your arms should be at your side with your palms pressing into the mat. With the feet flexed and the hands pressing, lift the chest and take several breaths.

4. Your gaze should be straight ahead with your eyes relaxed while taking these breaths.

5. It is helpful to think of your body as a "stick," strong and straight.

6. Feel your spine lifting out of the hips to elongate the back muscles. Breathe deeply to get oxygen into the cells of the muscles.

7. After three deep breaths, relax the pose and continue with the next pose.

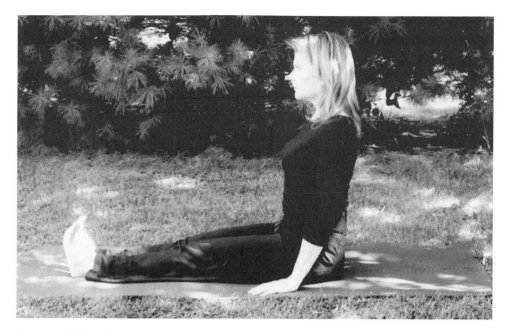

Figure 2.35 Stick Pose

Seated Forward Bend Pose

Seated Forward Bend Pose (Figure 2.36) is a good pose for calming anxiety. As the head reaches over the legs and the back lengthens, the mind and body are calmed. If your child is anxious or stressed, Seated Forward Bend Pose may provide an almost immediate sensation of calmness and tranquility.

This pose, although it looks like merely bending forward over the legs, may feel intense. The hamstrings and calves stretch. The back and shoulders also stretch as the body lowers over the legs.

This pose does not require excess strength or flexibility and may be modified as described below. Children with ASDs often do not like this pose at first. They think that the pose should be easy, because it looks like the person is just bending forward. However, the pose stretches all muscles from the feet to the top of the head. In addition, most people simply do not bend down and touch their toes regularly.

We suggest that you tell your child that he will probably feel many muscles stretching. He will also discover muscles that he may not know he even had. You can also have him notice that although the pose seems like only the legs should be stretching, the spine and back muscles are also stretching. We also suggest that you tell him that he should not force the pose. Rather, he needs to stop when he feels something in his body tense. At that point, he should take a deep breath. If, after this breath, he can move further, he should try to do so.

We usually explain to children that the goal of this pose is not to touch their toes, but to experience the pose. It is also suggested that you tell your child that although many people want to be the fastest and the best, yoga stresses getting to know yourself and your body. You are not in competition with anyone, not even yourself.

1. Come into a seated position at the back of your mat and stretch your legs out in front of you. Your legs may be relaxed, but should not flop out to the sides. The feet should be straight forward with a slight flex.

2. Bring in the abdomen slightly to help support your torso lift and lengthen upward.

3. Bring your arms over your head and gradually bend forward over your legs. Go as far down on your legs as possible. In time, as flexibility increases, you may be able to reach and clasp your feet.

4. Initially, you may modify the pose by only reaching your hands to your knees or shins (Figure 2.37).

5. At whatever place you have reached your hands, bring your chest up, and take a breath before you bend over into the forward bend. This breath will help you to remember to lengthen your body out toward the front wall, instead of rounding your chest into your body. The idea is to stretch out your spine and shoulders, as opposed to pulling your head down into your legs.

6. Now, lower your torso into a bend over your legs. Stay where you feel the stretch, but do not force the stretch. The stretch will increase in time. Think about breathing into your upper back and shoulders, to allow these areas to stretch further over the legs.

7. Take five breaths in this position. Think about relaxing your upper body onto your legs. When you are finished with the pose, slowly come up to a seated position.

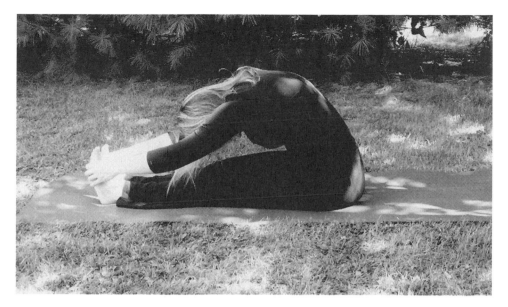

Figure 2.36 Seated Forward Bend Pose

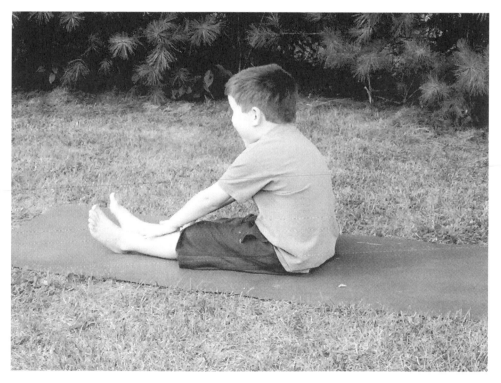

Figure 2.37 Modified Seated Forward Bend Pose

Spread Leg Forward Bend Pose

This pose (Figure 2.38) stretches the inner legs and hips. It also helps to stretch and elongate the spine and relax the whole torso. Although the movement is simple, the pose may be intense. The bending forward motion over the legs may feel stressful to many children, especially children who are not particularly active.

This pose, like Seated Forward Bend Pose, is also very calming when the head and torso are bent over the legs. Your child may use this pose and Seated Forward Bend to reduce anxiety. Feel free to encourage him to do this pose when feeling stressed during the day.

Like Seated Forward Bend Pose, this pose may be more difficult than it looks. Children with ASDs may be uncomfortable with the stretch in the inner thigh and groin area. We suggest that you remind your child that he should not force his body towards the floor. Additionally, remind him to tune into his body and listen to what it is "saying" to him. Explain to him that although the body cannot use words to speak, it communicates to our mind in other ways, such as with pain, anxiety, and feeling uncomfortable. Many people tend to ignore their bodies.

This pose may give your child the opportunity to feel what is happening in his legs, spine, and the rest of his body. You may mention this idea to him to begin the process of having him become aware of his body's feelings, and needs. If he can learn to care for his physical self, he can learn to alleviate stress and anxiety. Yoga can be an important part of his learning to take care of his body.

1. Sit at the back of your mat with your legs straight out in front of you.

2. Spread your legs as far apart as is comfortable into a straddle position. Do not reach the point of pain. You will feel a little stretch in the legs, but not too much discomfort. Your flexibility will increase over time.

3. Raise your arms over your head and take a deep breath while stretching upward.

4. Slowly begin to lower your torso in the middle of your spread legs. When you feel that you have lowered your torso as much as possible, stop, and put your hands, forearms, or elbows on the floor, depending on the extent of your flexibility.

5. Expand your chest and spine outward. It is more important to have your chest expand and lengthen than it is to be able to put your head on the floor. Take care not to round the neck into the chest to attempt to reach lower to the floor.

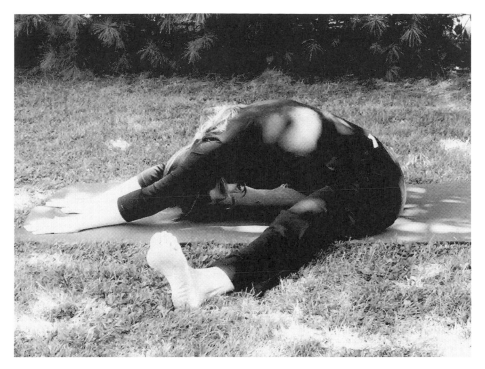

Figure 2.38 Spread Leg Forward Bend Pose

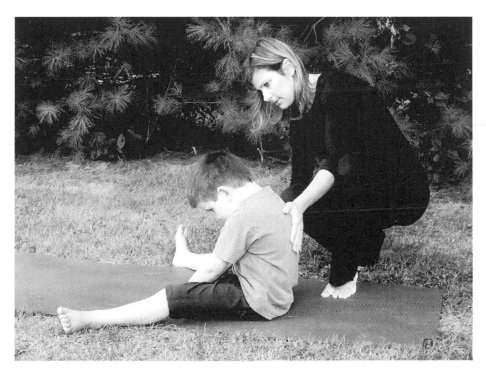

Figure 2.39 Modified Spread Leg Forward Bend Pose

6. If you cannot reach your forearms or elbows to the floor, keep your arms straight and press your palms into the floor (Figure 2.39).

7. Take several deep breaths and allow yourself to feel your inner legs stretching and releasing.

8. When you are finished with your breathing push up through your arms and bring your torso upright. With your hands around your thighs, slowly push your legs together and gently shake them to release the stretch.

Head-to-Knee Pose

Head-to-Knee Pose (Figure 2.40) is variation of the Seated Forward Bend Pose, in that the torso is being lowered over the leg. This pose will help to calm your child and alleviate tension. It also helps the spine elongate over the straight leg. It provides a slight spinal twist on both sides of the spine, depending on which leg is outstretched. Again, your child should only lower down over the leg as far as is comfortable.

The chest should be lengthened out towards the shin and foot, as opposed to folding in toward the knee. The bent leg may be bent in close to the thigh. A modification may be made by bending the leg to the other knee, as opposed to the thigh (Figure 2.41).

Because this pose is another version of forward bending, you may point out the idea of listening to your body and taking care of your body that was mentioned in the above two poses. The bent leg in this pose may cause some difficulty, many children often cannot bend forward as much as they think they should. We suggest that you remind your child to listen to his body and not force the stretch.

Often, the most difficult part of the yoga practice is to have the mind release all expectations about what should be and merely allow the body to let the poses happen. This concept is difficult to explain to children and others who are used to wanting to control their environment. Forward bending is a good introduction to the idea that to be comfortable in our body, you must allow your body to unfold on its own and not try to force your mind to rule your body.

1. Sit on the back of your mat and extend your legs out in front of you.

2. Slowly bend your right knee until your right heel is pressing into your left thigh. Your right heel should press firmly into your left thigh. If this is not comfortable, press your right heel lower onto your left thigh or near your left knee.

3. Try to keep both hips on the floor, to allow for some hip opening and to keep your balance.

4. Raise your arms over your head and stretch both arms toward the sky.

5. Slowly lower your outstretched arms over your right leg as far as possible.

6. Keep your chest and head reaching toward your right foot to lengthen the torso.

7. When you have determined how far you may comfortably stretch, place your arms, palms, or forearms on either side of your outstretched leg.

8. Hold this pose for three breaths. Try to feel your spine lengthening and your upper body both relaxing and stretching into the ground.

9. Slowly bring your torso up and sit upright. Put your legs out in front of you. Do the pose on the other side.

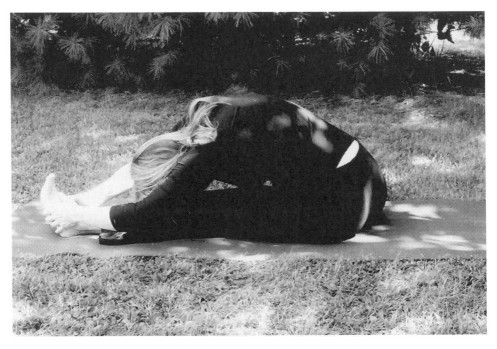

Figure 2.40 Head-to-Knee Pose

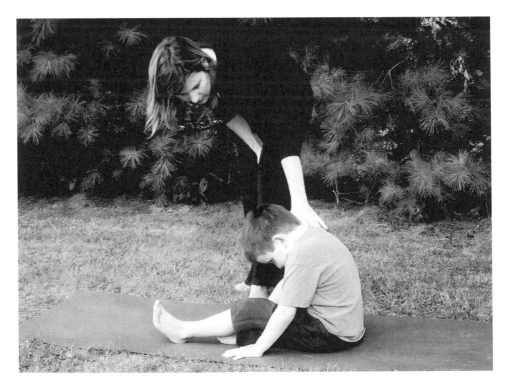

Figure 2.41 Modified Head-to-Knee Pose

Butterfly Pose

Butterfly Pose (Figure 2.42) opens the hips. It lengthens the spine and relaxes the shoulders. This pose does not require much muscle strength, but if the hips are very tight, the pose may be uncomfortable at first. In order to make your child more comfortable, yoga blocks may be placed under the knees. This supports the legs and allows the hip and groin area to stretch open gradually. Additionally, a pillow can be used with blocks to raise the hips to make the child more comfortable.

Surprisingly, many children with ASDs do not have a hard time with the hips opening. However, they often do not enjoy sitting on the floor because of low muscle tone and difficulty sitting up straight. In addition, the soles of the feet do not have to touch entirely. Often a child is only able to have the heels touch. It is best if your child is comfortable in the position, as it is helpful to have your child stay a little longer in this pose to allow the hips and groin to soften and release accumulated tension.

This pose gives a great feeling of freedom throughout the entire body. Much tension is stored in the hip joints. Many yogis believe that unresolved emotions from physical and emotional traumas are stored in the hip area. By releasing this area, both the body and mind may feel freer, lighter, and less encumbered. Children with ASDs often have a hard time with daily living due to the symptoms of their disorder. Because they often have difficulty expressing themselves to others, these kids may internalize their daily stresses. This pose may help kids with ASDs release the stress in their bodies.

Children with ASDs understand the idea of Butterfly Pose. They are often relieved that the forward bending is over. They often feel "all wrung out" and "really relaxed" at this point in the yoga practice.

We suggest that you tell your child to close his eyes and imagine that his legs are opening like beautiful butterfly wings. Tell your child to imagine that his breath is opening the wings of the butterfly and allowing all the old energy to release. His breath brings in new, fresh energy into the body. Although children may think that it is "weird" to think about the butterfly image, they can benefit from using such a visualization. Do not be afraid to make up stories or images to assist your child in getting into and staying in the yoga poses. These images will undoubtedly stay with your child and make the yoga practice more interesting.

1. Sit at the back of your mat with your legs outstretched and take a deep breath.

2. Slowly bend your legs and bring the soles of your feet together in front of your groin. Bring your feet as close as possible to your groin. Take care not to strain your knees while bringing your feet together. Only bring your feet as close to your groin as is comfortable.

3.   Try to bring the soles of your feet together. Do not worry if your heels do not touch.

4.   You may need to place a block under each knee to help support your legs and to ease the stretch on your hips (Figure 2.43).

5.   Grasp your feet with both hands and sit as erect as possible while inhaling. You will feel your spine elongate and your chest expand as you take a breath.

6.   Take three breaths. Try to concentrate on feeling the hips open from the weight of gravity pressing on your legs. After your hips become more open, the blocks may be removed to allow for more hip opening.

7.   Eventually, you may be able to grasp your feet around the top and open your feet as you would open a book, allowing for a fuller opening in the hips. For the beginner, this step may be omitted.

8.   Use your breath to relax your body and try to imagine that the tight areas in the hips are receiving support from your breath. You may tell your child to imagine that any tightness is being lifted off the hips and out of the body like floating balloons each time he exhales. Eventually the hips will soften and release and he will experience the extremely freeing feeling that comes from the hip opening poses.

9.   After you are finished with the breaths, slowly straighten your legs in front of you and take several deep breaths. Allow your body to relax before continuing with the next pose.

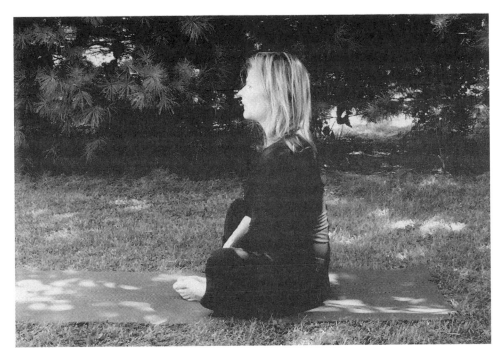

Figure 2.42 Butterfly Pose

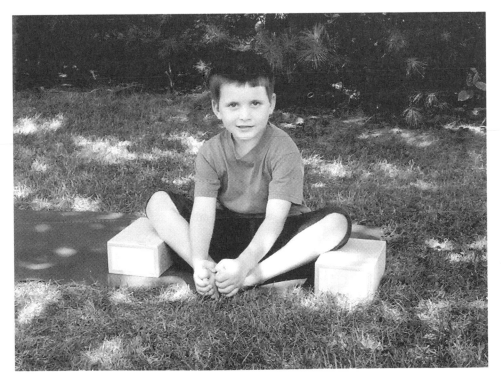

Figure 2.43 Modified Butterfly Pose

Reclining Butterfly Pose

This pose (Figure 2.44) continues to open the hips and release the spine. Some children may find this pose easier than Butterfly Pose because the hips have already begun to be open and they are already somewhat warmed. Additionally, your child may find this pose more comfortable because the body is in the supine position. The pose does not involve much abdominal or torso strength.

Your child should be encouraged to breathe into his hips and try to release any tension that may have accumulated in his body. Children with ASDs often enjoy this pose compared to the more physically challenging poses. Your child may be encouraged to stay in the pose longer than three breaths if he so desires.

Children are often surprised at how gravity presses the hips down when they are lying on their backs. They find that once they are relaxed into this pose, they are more comfortable than when the muscles are tensed. It is suggested that you help your child relax by encouraging him to breathe into his hip areas. You can help him visualize that the area is releasing many small butterflies that flutter upward toward the sky with each exhalation. If the hips are tight, you may place the yoga blocks underneath each thigh for support.

1. Lie on your back on the mat with your body relaxed. Have your arms by your sides and your eyes closed. Take several deep breaths.

2. Bend your knees out to the sides of your body and bring the soles of your feet together.

3. Bring the soles of your feet as far up towards the groin as possible, but do not strain. Only bring the soles of the feet as far towards the groin as is comfortable. Feel your hips open and relax.

4. Stretch your arms over your head. Take three deep breaths, feeling your hips opening while your arms are stretching and your torso is lengthening. Try to keep your lower back pressed into the ground, and do not let the spine arch. Feel the various places in your body that may be releasing, especially the hips, spine, and shoulders.

5. After you have taken three or more breaths, slowly straighten your legs. Bring your arms to your sides, and rest for a moment, concentrating on the feeling in your hips.

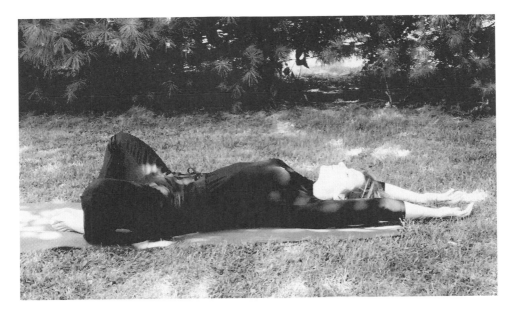

Figure 2.44 Reclining Butterfly Pose

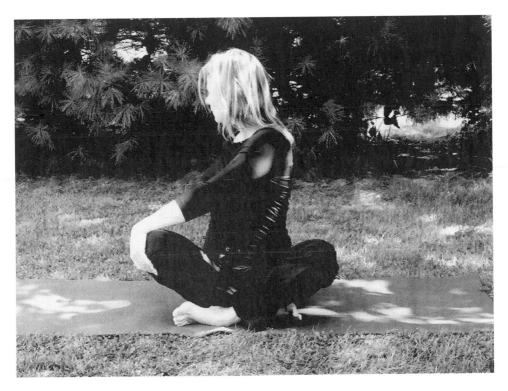

Figure 2.45 Seated Spinal Twist Pose

Seated Spinal Twist Pose

Twists are very beneficial in keeping the spine fluid and supple. Spinal twists move the body in an unusual way and this movement may help alleviate stress in areas of the body that are usually hidden and forgotten. Twists help to relieve congestion in the internal organs by bringing fresh oxygen to them, and by squeezing and releasing these organs. Spinal twists are similar to a massage for your organs.

Since these poses will be unfamiliar to your child, they should be demonstrated to him first. Additionally, you will want to physically guide him into the pose to make sure he will be comfortable sitting in the pose on his own. The twisting poses will help him explore new feelings in his body in a comfortable manner.

Children with ASDs are often very uncomfortable with the idea of twisting their bodies. We suggest that you remind your child that he will be safe and that you are there to guide him. It is not recommended that you tell him the benefits of the pose as described above. We worry that he would get fixated on visions of internal organs being twisted like a wrung out towel! It is beneficial to merely guide him into the position and have him try the twist. At first, children are somewhat uncomfortable. However, they then usually relax and stop complaining.

1. Sit cross-legged at the front of your mat. Straighten your spine and lift the crown of your head to the sky. Lengthen your torso as much as possible, so that when you twist you are not grinding down into your body. Instead, you are freeing the spine by lengthening and twisting.

2. Begin to twist to the right by placing your right hand behind your back as far as possible. Keep the right hand on the floor and try to press into the palm to keep the spine lifted upward.

3. Place your left hand on your right knee to help your body go into the twist. Do not push your body farther than is comfortable.

4. Take a breath in, and think about lengthening your body upward to the sky. Exhale and slowly twist your body to the right.

5. When you are "twisted," take three breaths in this position. Feel your spine twist and stretch (Figure 2.45).

6. You may look over your right shoulder towards the back of the room, but you should not feel tension in your neck. If you cannot look backward, then keep your neck in whatever position is comfortable while you hold the twist.

7. After holding this position for three breaths, release the pose and sit cross-legged for a few breaths. Then repeat the twist to the left side.

Easy Spinal Twist Pose

Easy Spinal Twist is, as the name implies, an "easier" pose than Seated Spinal Twist, because your child is lying on the mat rather than sitting in a cross-legged position (Figure 2.46). This pose is still very effective for releasing the spine, massaging the organs, and releasing tension from the body. Your child may feel tightness in the pose at the beginning, because the pose involves twisting the spine in an unfamiliar movement but, with practice, he may welcome the tension release associated with this pose.

Many children with ASDs enjoy this pose. Initially they do not realize that this is another twisting position. Some children say that their arms outstretched "feels really good." They are often glad that they get to lie down on the mat. We suggest that you tell your child that he is near the end of the practice and how open and stress-free his body should feel. It is important that he realizes that anxiety and tension are not constant physical and emotion feelings that he must endure. Part of the importance of yoga is teaching your child to relieve his own pain, tension, and stress.

1. Lie on the mat on your back with your arms by your sides and your body relaxed.

2. Extend your arms out to the sides so they are straight out from the shoulders. Your arms will form the letter "T" with your torso.

3. Slowly bend the right leg and place the sole of your foot on your left knee.

4. Make sure that your shoulders stay as close to the floor as possible. Slowly move the bent right leg to the left. Your body will want to fall over the left side, but try to keep your shoulders on the floor.

5. Keep your left leg as straight as possible. Additionally, keep the left foot flexed, if possible, and the leg pressing into the floor. This way the body feels grounded, even though it is twisting.

6. Move your head to the left, so that your left cheek is resting on the floor.

7. Take three deep breaths into the pose. Try to release any tight spots in your body or tension you may feel by inhaling deeply. Imagine the breath going into the tight area, and then release tension upon exhalation.

8. Slowly bring your knee upright and then release your legs and stretch them out for a moment.

9. Repeat the position on your left side.

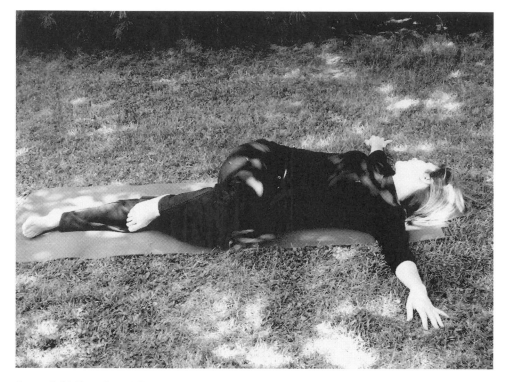

Figure 2.46 Easy Spinal Twist Pose

Child's Pose

Child's Pose (Figure 2.47) should always be practiced as the second to last pose, with Corpse Pose being the last pose of the practice. Child's Pose may also be used as a resting pose between postures if your child needs extra time to rejuvenate or relax before going onto the next posture. Child's Pose stretches the upper back and spine and also relaxes the whole body.

This pose releases all the muscles and allows the body to relax into the floor. In addition, the forehead is pressed into the mat and this slight pressure relaxes the head. Many children find this pose very peaceful and look forward to ending the practice with this pose. This pose is also a good way for your child to calm down or relax whenever he is agitated, or even before bed to help him get to sleep.

There have been many nights when Stacey has done this pose in bed and felt relaxed and quieted enough to fall asleep. This pose does not require much strength or flexibility and most children feel confident performing it. The idea is that the pose is like a child folding himself up and burrowing into himself to provide self-nurture.

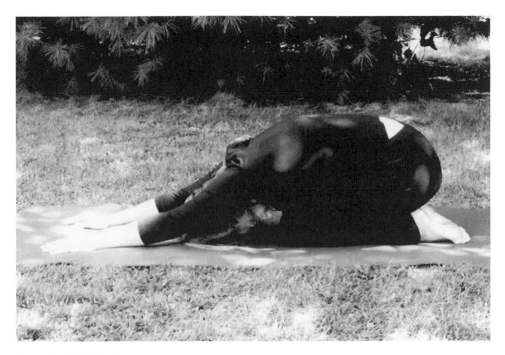

Figure 2.47 Child's Pose

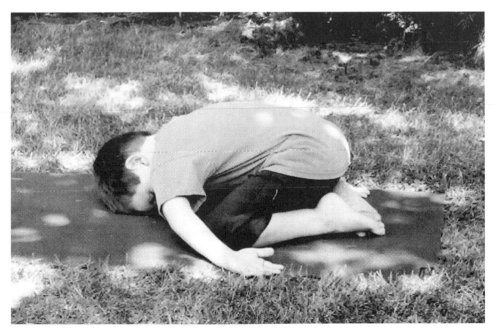

Figure 2.48 Modified Child's Pose

This pose gives a sense of calm and quiet that your child may never have felt before. He may remain in this pose for longer than the usual three breaths to allow his body and mind to relax. As a modification, the knees may be spread and the belly may rest in the space between the knees, if this position is more comfortable for him. Additionally, he may place his arms at his sides rather than lift them overhead if this is more comfortable.

Child's Pose is often favored by children with ASDs. It helps individuals shut out the world for a moment. Children love the feeling of being safe and secure. Rubbing your child's back while they are in this position can help increase feelings of security and bliss. It is suggested that you mention to your child that this pose can help him get to sleep or to relax after a stressful day. We have found that linking yoga poses with daily life helps children view yoga as a method to be able to help, as opposed to being simply extra work.

1. Lay on your belly on the mat with your arms by your sides. Take a deep breath and relax.

2. Slowly push yourself up until you are on your hands and knees. Your arms should be directly below your shoulders. Pause here a moment and take a deep breath. Try not to let your shoulders sag into your back. Try to look like you are getting ready to crawl.

3. Lower your buttocks onto your heels and pause.

4. Lower your chest onto the knees with your arms stretched in front of you.

5. If necessary, you may spread your knees and place your belly into the space between your knees.

6. You may also rest your arms by the sides if having your arms overhead is uncomfortable (Figure 2.48).

7. Place your forehead on the floor and relax your body. You should feel a stretch in your upper back as your body relaxes into the earth.

8. Take several breaths and then push out of this position and lie on your back on your mat to prepare for the next pose.

Corpse Pose

This pose (Figure 2.49) should always be the last pose of each yoga practice. It has several benefits. It is a total relaxation pose. This means that it allows the body and mind to totally relax and let go. The other important aspect of this pose is that it allows the body and the nervous systems to absorb all the benefits of the previous poses. Corpse Pose gives the body a chance to pause between the yoga practice and reentering the regular world and to rest with no pressures or worries. Because the world may be such a stressful, uncertain, and uncontrollable place for a child with an ASD, Corpse Pose may provide a brief respite from pressures.

Your child should envision his body sinking into the ground with all physical and emotional tension seeping out of his body. The breath should be deep and smooth and he may think about how his breath feels entering and leaving his body while his body is still.

This pose may be held for two to fifteen minutes. Although children may like the idea that they do not have to "do" anything in this pose, they usually find that it is difficult to be still. Your child may want to finish yoga practice already and play. However, this pose is important because it will help him experience what it feels like to stop moving and to take a break without distractions. A timer set for one minute during this pose is suggested to show him when the session will end.

Eye bags are particularly useful for this pose. They block out visual distractions and stimulation and increase the feeling of calm. Place the eye bag over your child's eyes once he has settled into this pose.

1. Lay on your mat on your back with your arms by your side. Your arms should be slightly out from the sides of your body.

2. Your legs should be outstretched and relaxed. Have the length of about one foot between your feet.

3. Keep your feet relaxed. They should not be either pointed or flexed, but instead remain in a neutral position.

4. Your head should be relaxed, but aligned with the spine.

5. Your torso and spine should be in a straight line on the floor.

6. Take several deep breaths in this position and allow your body to release and relax.

7. Next, tense and release each part of your body to experience a sense of deep relaxation and enjoyment. Start at your feet and tense the muscles of your feet and tocs. Hold for a moment then relax.

8. Continue this exercise by then tensing and releasing the following: your legs and thighs, your abdomen and chest, your arms, your hands and fingers, and finally your face and neck.

9. After you are finished tensing and releasing the various parts of your body, tense and release the entire body and then lay quietly for about five minutes to rest and rejuvenate.

10. After you are finished with Corpse Pose, stand up from your mat. You are now ready to face the rest of the day with vigor, calmness, and energy!

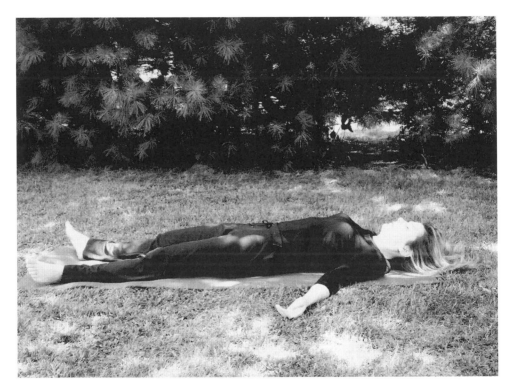

Figure 2.49 Corpse Pose

3: Yogic Breathing

Proper breathing is an important part of yogic philosophy. Yogis feel that good breathing is a way to purify and cleanse the body and mind. Different types of breathing exercises may also balance the nerves and all the systems of the body. Whole books have been devoted to the benefits and techniques of different types of yogic breathing.

For this guide, we have chosen several different breathing practices that can balance the body systems, enhance abdominal strength, and relieve the body of tension. Learning different ways to breathe is important for a child with an Autism Spectrum Disorder (ASD). Bringing awareness to the breath helps your child to bring awareness to his body.

After your child has gained some insight into how body movements coordinate, he may then begin to understand how he may control his body. He will begin to perceive how he may physically interact with the environment in a way that is safe and less stressful. Breath awareness brings instant recognition of how the mind and body are connected. Breath awareness may also be very grounding. An awareness of breath brings your child into his body immediately.

Ancient yogis developed special breathing methods. They are still very relevant and important to learn today. Children with ASDs have a lot to benefit from using such methods.

It is best to explain to your child that the breathing exercise will help him to be calm and feel rejuvenated. You can also explain that some of the exercises can help with feelings of anger, and they may be used at any time.

Ujjayi Breathing

Ujjayi Breathing is the usual breath that is taught and used during yoga practice. Ujjayi Breathing makes a small sound with each breath, so by listening to this breath during the yoga practice, this sound may become a kind of meditation while doing yoga poses.

This breath technique helps to keep the breath slow and steady and helps to ensure that there is a steady supply of oxygen to the muscles during the yoga practice. This breath only uses the nose, so the air is warmed and cleaned. Ujjayi

Breathing also helps your child to resist panting or tensing in harder poses, as the breathing method is slow and deep.

1. To practice this technique, sit cross-legged or in any comfortable position on your mat.

2. Take a breath through your nose with your mouth closed. Try to make and hear a sound like the ocean when you inhale. You may need to slightly constrict the opening in the front of your throat to make this sound. You may point to the hollow in the base of your throat to show your child where the throat restriction should be.

4. Exhale slowly through the nose. When exhaling with this breathing method, you should hear the same ocean sound.

5. Keep your breath slow and deep. Practice this breath for several moments. When your child gains proficiency with the yoga poses, you may encourage your child to incorporate Ujjayi Breathing into any of the poses.

Skull Shining Breath

Skull Shining Breath uses the abdominal muscles. This breath invigorates the entire body while it uses the lower belly muscles. By practicing this breathing exercise, your child becomes aware of using the belly muscles rather than the chest muscles to breathe. When the belly is used to breathe, the belly expands, allowing more air to enter the belly and chest.

This breathing technique may become tiresome for the abdominal muscles, so no more than twenty repetitions for the beginner are recommended. When the abdominal muscles become stronger, up to fifty repetitions may be done.

1. Sit on your mat in a cross-legged position with your hands resting in your lap.

2. Take a regular inhalation through your nose.

3. Then make a sharp, strong exhalation through your nose. Your belly muscles should help you make this exhalation sharp, fast, and strong.

4. Take a small inhalation through your nose and then make another sharp exhalation.

5. Try to feel your stomach muscles working with each exhale. Think of the belly as a bellows that helps to expel all the air in the body out through the nose.

6.   Repeat from twenty to fifty times and then relax. You should feel energy and aliveness throughout your body.

Curled Tongue Breath

This breath helps to release anger and frustration (Figure 3.1). Your child may only perform this breath if he can curl his tongue. If he cannot curl his tongue, he should skip this breathing exercise and practice Lion Breath to release anger. It helps if your child imagines that he is breathing in clear, fresh air through his curled tongue and that he is expelling old, stale, angry air. The tongue acts a funnel for the anger to be dispelled. The inhalation and exhalation should be as long and slow as possible.

1.   Sit cross-legged on your mat with your arms resting comfortably on your legs.

2.   Curl your tongue.

3.   Slowly breathe air in through your curled tongue. The air will feel cool on your tongue. Try to inhale to a count of eight.

4.   Try to breathe the air down into the belly as opposed to holding the air in your chest.

5.   Slowly begin to exhale through your curled tongue to a count of eight. Try to get your belly empty of all air. Imagine all your anger is being blown out of the body through your curled tongue.

6.   Repeat three times.

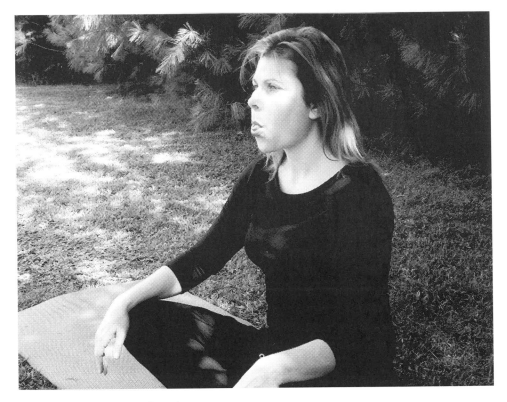

Figure 3.1 Curled Tongue Breath

Lion Breath

Lion Breath helps to make energy move through the body (Figure 3.2). It also helps to expel anger and resentment. This is a good breath to use if your child is having difficulty in releasing feelings. Your child should think about what his problem is, and do several Lion Breaths to get the problem and the negative feelings out of his system.

It is helpful if you demonstrate Lion Breath first, and then actually do the breathing exercise with your child. This breath technique is extremely freeing and cleansing, and the results are felt immediately.

1. Sit on your mat in a kneeling position. Your legs may be together or slightly apart.

2. Your arms should be relaxed and your hands may rest on your lap.

3. Open your mouth wide. Point your tongue as far out of your mouth as possible.

4.   With your mouth open, make a roaring sound. Feel the air and energy move out of your mouth from deep within your belly. Keep roaring until you feel that you want to stop.

5.   Take a deep breath and then do three more Lion Breaths. Each time you practice one of these breaths, visualize all anger, resentment, and rage coming loose from inside your body and being expelled out of your mouth. Children will probably like this exercise once they become accustomed to it.

At first, your child may seem a little disturbed when he watches you model this breath. When he actually tries Lion Breath, however, he will surely like the feeling and sound of being a lion.

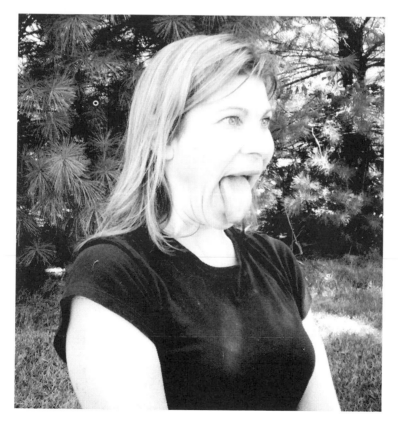

Figure 3.2 Lion Breath

Alternate Nostril Breathing

Alternate Nostril Breathing (Figure 3.3) is a breathing technique that is used to balance the nervous system. It is not difficult to do, but will be very different from anything that your child has ever done before. In addition, it seems very "yoga like" because the finger position will feel foreign at first. This breathing exercise has been included because of its effectiveness. Your child should be encouraged to become familiar with this technique, in spite of its strangeness.

Visualizations go very well with this breathing technique. Guide your child through the breathing along with the visualization. To start Alternate Nostril Breathing, he should be breathing in air from the left nostril with the right nostril closed (using his own thumb). He may be helped to envision the sunlight, in the form of rainbow colors, coming from the sky and streaming into his body with his breath. You will then have him close both nostrils. Help him envision the rainbow energy swirling inside his body to give his body heat and strength and to enliven all parts of his body.

Then he may let his breath out of the right nostril. He may imagine that the exhalation is a pale shade of gray, and that the exhale is expelling all the old, tired energy that was in his body. What is left in his body is the fresh new rainbow energy that will give him new ideas and actions. He inhales through his right nostril. This nostril brings the calmer, serene moon energy into the body.

You then may help him imagine a rush of light blue energy coming into his body. The pale blue represents the pale moon energy that calms and soothes. As he inhales, he should imagine this energy coming from the moon and entering his body. While he is holding his breath, he should think about the blue swirl reaching all parts of his body and making him calm and serene. When he exhales out of his left nostril, he should envision all anxiety and tension leaving his body on a blue trail of light. This breathing method can help a child anywhere, for instance at school.

1. Sit cross-legged or in any comfortable position at the front of your mat.

2. Using your right hand, fold the first two fingers under your thumb, so only your last two fingers are sticking up (Figure 3.4).

3. Place your thumb on your right nostril and close this nostril.

4. Slowly inhale for a count of three to five through your left nostril. Use the visualization of inhaling sun energy into your body.

5. Close your left nostril with the fourth finger of your right hand and hold the breath for a count of three to five. Imagine rainbow energy swirling around in your body.

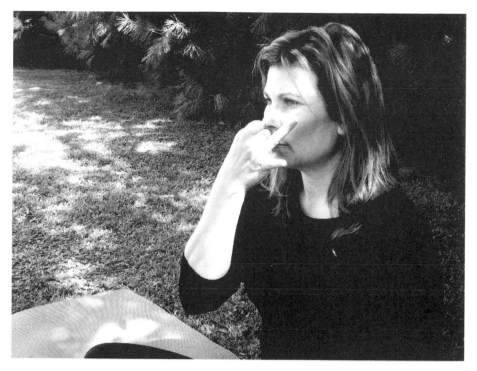

Figure 3.3 Alternate Nostril Breathing

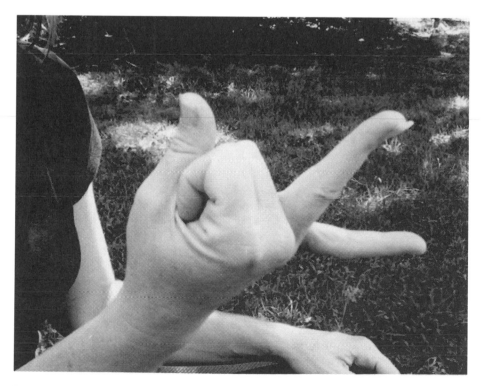

Figure 3.4 Alternate Nostril Breathing Hand Position

6. Open your right nostril by releasing your thumb and exhale for a count of three (or up to five), releasing the energy that was swirling in your body.

7. Inhale through the right nostril for a count of three (or up to five) and imagine a blue stream of energy from the moon is entering the body.

8. Put your thumb back on your right nostril and let the energy swirl around in your body for three to five counts.

9. Release your fourth finger from your left nostril and let the air stream out of that nostril, releasing toxins.

10. This is one round of alternate nostril breathing. You may stop here or do one or two more rounds. Concentrate on how your body and mind is feeling when you are finished.

4: Shorter Yoga Sequences

There are times when you may not have time to do the full yoga session outlined above. Possibly, your child may feel tired or weak, or does not want to practice yoga on a given day. Instead of completely avoiding the yoga practice, consider trying one of the shorter yoga sequences outlined below. These sequences, although abbreviated, are still very beneficial. The shorter sequences help your child stay supple and flexible. In addition, it is important to practice consistently to get the full benefit of yoga practice.

It is better to practice three times per week for ten minutes than to practice a full forty-five minute session once a week. In addition, it will help keep your child's practice consistent if he knows he cannot get out of the exercises just because he may not "feel like it." We grouped some of the poses that we feel flow well together. You do not have to adhere strictly to the exact poses or the sequence of poses. However, end each session with Child's Pose and Corpse Pose for final stretching and relaxation.

Short sequence 1

Cat Pose

Mountain Pose

Spinal Rolls

Downward Dog Pose

Warrior II Pose

Stick Pose

Butterfly Pose

Lion Breath

Child's Pose

Corpse Pose

Short sequence 2

Sitting Pose

Shoulder Opener Pose

Mountain Pose

Chair Pose

Triangle Pose

Downward Dog Pose

Tree Pose

Sphinx Pose

Seated Forward Bend Pose

Seated Spinal Twist Pose

Child's Pose

Corpse Pose

References

Bernardi, L., Sleight, P., Bandinelli, G., Cencetti, S., Fattorini, L., Wdowczyc-Szulc, J., and Lagi, A. (2001) "Effect of rosary prayer and yoga mantras on autonomic cardiovascular rhythms: comparative study." *British Medical Journal*, December 22–29, 323 (7327), pp.1446–1449.

Khanam, A. A., Sachdeva, U., Guleria, R., and Deepak, K. K. (1996) "Study of pulmonary and autonomic functions of asthma patients after yoga training." *Indian Journal of Physiology and Pharmacology*, October 40(4), pp.318–324.

Naveen, K. V., Nagarathna R., Nagendra, H. R., and Telles, S. (1997) "Yoga breathing through a particular nostril increases spatial memory scores without lateralized effects." *Psychology Reports*, October 81(2), pp.555–561.

Panjwani, W., Selvamurthy, W., Singh, S. H., Gupta, H. L., Thakur, L., and Rai, U. C. (1997) "Effect of Sahaja yoga practice on seizure control and EEG changes in patients of epilepsy." *Indian Journal of Medical Research*, March 103, pp.165–172.

Shannahoff-Khalsa, D. and Beckett, L. R. (1996) "Clinical case report: efficacy of yogic techniques in the treatment of obsessive compulsive disorders." *International Journal of Neuroscience*, March 85(1–2), pp.1–17.

Telles, S., Hanumanthaiah, B., Nagarathna, R., and Nagendra, H. R. (1993) "Improvement in static motor performance following yogic training of school children." *Perceptual and Motor Skills*, April 38(2), pp.143–144.